Unicompartmental Knee Arthroplasty: The Modern Frontier

Editors

KEVIN D. PLANCHER
STEPHANIE C. PETTERSON

CLINICS IN SPORTS MEDICINE

www.sportsmed.theclinics.com

Consulting Editor
MARK D. MILLER

January 2014 • Volume 33 • Number 1

ELSEVIER

1600 John F. Kennedy Boulevard • Suite 1800 • Philadelphia, Pennsylvania, 19103-2899

http://www.theclinics.com

CLINICS IN SPORTS MEDICINE Volume 33, Number 1
January 2014 ISSN 0278-5919, ISBN-13: 978-0-323-22740-7

Editor: Jennifer Flynn-Briggs

Clinics in Sports Medicine (ISSN 0278-5919) is published quarterly by Elsevier Inc., 360 Park Avenue South, New York, NY 10010-1710. Months of issue are January, April, July, and October. Business and Editorial Offices: 1600 John F. Kennedy Blvd., Ste. 1800, Philadelphia, PA 19103-2899. Customer Service Office: 3251 Riverport Lane, Maryland Heights, MO 63043. Periodicals postage paid at New York, NY and additional mailing offices. Subscription prices are $340.00 per year (US individuals), $540.00 per year (US institutions), $165.00 per year (US students), $385.00 per year (Canadian individuals), $666.00 per year (Canadian institutions), $235.00 (Canadian students), $470.00 per year (foreign individuals), $666.00 per year (foreign institutions), and $235.00 per year (foreign students). Foreign air speed delivery is included in all *Clinics* subscription prices. All prices are subject to change without notice. **POSTMASTER:** Send address changes to *Clinics in Sports Medicine*, Elsevier Health Sciences Division, Subscription Customer Service, 3251 Riverport Lane, Maryland Heights, MO 63043. Customer Service (orders, claims, online, change of address): Elsevier Health Sciences Division, Subscription Customer Service, 3251 Riverport Lane, Maryland Heights, MO 63043. Tel: 1-800-654-2452 (U.S. and Canada); 314-447-8871 (outside U.S. and Canada). Fax: 314-447-8029. E-mail: journalscustomerservice-usa@elsevier.com (for print support); journalsonlinesupport-usa@elsevier.com (for online support).

Reprints. For copies of 100 or more of articles in this publication, please contact the Commercial Reprints Department, Elsevier Inc., 360 Park Avenue South, New York, NY 10010-1710. Tel.: 212-633-3874; Fax: 212-633-3820; E-mail: reprints@elsevier.com.

Clinics in Sports Medicine is covered in *MEDLINE/PubMed (Index Medicus) Current Contents/Clinical Medicine, Excerpta Medica,* and *ISI/Biomed.*

Printed and bound by CPI Group (UK) Ltd, Croydon, CR0 4YY

Transferred to digital print 2013

Contributors

CONSULTING EDITOR

MARK D. MILLER, MD
S. Ward Casscells Professor of Orthopaedic Surgery, University of Virginia; Team Physician, James Madison University, JBJS Deputy Editor for Sports Medicine; Director, Miller Review Course, Charlottesville, Virginia

EDITORS

KEVIN D. PLANCHER, MD, MS, FACS, FAAOS
Associate Clinical Professor, Department of Orthopaedics, Albert Einstein College of Medicine, Plancher Orthopaedics and Sports Medicine, New York, New York; Fellowship Director, Orthopaedic Foundation for Active Lifestyles, Greenwich, Connecticut

STEPHANIE C. PETTERSON, PhD
Director of Research, Orthopaedic Foundation for Active Lifestyles, Greenwich, Connecticut

ASSOCIATE EDITOR

ALBERT S.M. DUNN, DO
Fellow, Department of Orthopaedics, Orthopaedic Foundation for Active Lifestyles, Greenwich, Connecticut

AUTHORS

AHMAD BADRI, DO
Associate Professor, Touro COM, Harlem, New York; Department of Orthopedics, Jersey City Medical Center, Jersey City; Department of Orthopedics, Meadowlands Hospital Medical Center, Secaucus, New Jersey

KEITH R. BEREND, MD
Associate, Joint Implant Surgeon Inc, New Albany, Ohio

JACK M. BERT, MD
Minnesota Bone and Joint Specialists, Ltd, St Paul, Minnesota

TIMOTHY M. BERT, MD
Hedley Orthopedic Clinic, Phoenix, Arizona

JOEL L. BOYD, MD
TRIA Orthopaedic Center, Bloomington, Minnesota

JOSEPH BURKHARDT, DO
Clinical Professor, Michigan State University, East Lansing, Michigan; Department of Orthopedics, Bronsone Battle Creek Hospital, Bronson, Battle, Michigan

MARCO KAWAMURA DEMANGE, MD, PhD
Attending Orthopedic Surgeon, Department of Orthopedic Surgery and Traumatology, University of São Paulo, São Paulo, São Paulo, Brazil; Post-Doctoral Research Fellow, Hospital for Special Surgery, Weil Cornell Medical College, New York, New York

ALBERT S.M. DUNN, DO
Fellow, Department of Orthopaedics, Orthopaedic Foundation for Active Lifestyles, Greenwich, Connecticut

JASON M. HURST, MD
Associate, Joint Implant Surgeon Inc, New Albany, Ohio

CHAD A. KURTENBACH, MD
TRIA Orthopaedic Center, Bloomington, Minnesota

BRETT LEVINE, MD, MS
Assistant Professor and Residency Program Director, Rush University Medical Center, Chicago, Illinois

ANTHONY MINIACI, MD, FRCSC
Professor of Surgery, Cleveland Clinic Lerner College of Medicine, Cleveland Clinic, Garfield Heights, Ohio

BRIAN T. PALUMBO, MD
Adult Reconstruction Fellow, Harvard Combined Orthopaedics, Brigham and Women's Hospital, Boston, Massachusetts

STEPHANIE C. PETTERSON, PhD
Director of Research, Orthopaedic Foundation for Active Lifestyles, Greenwich, Connecticut

KEVIN D. PLANCHER, MD, MS, FACS, FAAOS
Associate Clinical Professor, Department of Orthopaedics, Albert Einstein College of Medicine; Plancher Orthopaedics and Sports Medicine, New York, New York; Fellowship Director, Orthopaedic Foundation for Active Lifestyles, Greenwich, Connecticut

ANDREW J. RIFF, MD
Section of Adult Reconstruction, Department of Orthopaedic Surgery, Rush University Medical Center, Chicago, Illinois

MARTIN ROCHE, MD
Holy Cross Orthopedic Institute, Lauderdale, Florida

SCOTT RODEO, MD
Attending Orthopedic Surgeon, Hospital for Special Surgery, Professor of Orthopaedic Surgery, Weil Cornell Medical College, New York, New York

AARON G. ROSENBERG, MD
Professor of Orthopaedic Surgery, Director of Adult Reconstruction, Rush University Medical Center, Chicago, Illinois

ALEXANDER P. SAH, MD
Private Practice, Institute for Joint Restoration, Washington Hospital, Fremont, California

RICHARD D. SCOTT, MD
Professor of Orthopaedic Surgery, Harvard Medical School, Boston, Massachusetts

ROBBY S. SIKKA, MD
TRIA Orthopaedic Center, Bloomington, Minnesota

MARCO SISTO, BA
Research Fellow, Hospital for Special Surgery, Weil Cornell Medical College, New York, New York

ALAN VALADIE, MD
Medical Director, The Joint Center at Blake Medical Center; Coastal Orthopedics and Sports Medicine, Bradenton, Florida

CRAIG J. DELLA VALLE, MD
Associate Professor, Section of Adult Reconstruction, Department of Orthopaedic Surgery, Rush University Medical Center, Chicago, Illinois

Contents

and the native knee and recent evidence showing excellent survivorship and functionality, UKA is an excellent alternative to TKA in the appropriate patient. This article discusses the use of intramedullary guides for preparation in partial knee replacement surgery. The concerns of complications arising from cannulating the medullary canal and excessive bleeding have not been seen. The intramedullary UKA yields high levels of success and long-term outcomes, with excellent alignment.

With the recent increase in medial unicompartmental arthroplasty, this article reviews the design history, indications, results, and modern technique for the implantation of the Oxford mobile-bearing unicompartmental arthroplasty. The article also discusses how the indications for the Oxford differ from the historical indications for medial unicompartmental arthroplasty and supports this paradigm shift with review of the recent data. A detailed series of surgical pearls is also presented to help surgeons with the surgical nuances of the Oxford partial knee.

Since its introduction, unicompartmental knee arthroplasty has been controversial because of poor early clinical outcomes due to implant design, bony fixation, surgical instrumentation, and technique. Improvements in surgical technique and implant design have resulted in improved outcomes and greater survivorship. The ability to optimize a patient's surgical result requires appropriate patient selection, and the ability to accurately achieve your surgical plan. Implant placement, limb alignment, soft tissue balance, joint line preservation, and joint stability are the critical factors in obtaining a successful outcome.

In the past decade, there has been a major increase in the use of unicompartmental knee arthroplasty (UKA) as surgical techniques have been refined and patient selection has improved. UKAs now account for 8% to 10% of knee arthoplasty procedures. Recent studies have suggested excellent medium- and long-term results of UKA. Overall, results have shown 85% to 90% survivorship at 10 years, with 90% of patients reporting good to excellent subjective and objective outcomes. Recent studies suggest that unicompartmental arthroplasty allows a high percentage of patients to return to pre-operative sport and activity participation.

Unicompartmental knee arthroplasty has experienced resurgence in popularity because of the lower morbidity of the procedure and the proposed benefits over total knee replacement in appropriately selected patients.

Improved component designs and advanced surgical techniques have promoted excellent results. Expanded indications to include the very young and the elderly have yielded comparable clinical outcomes. Nonetheless, the success of unicompartmental replacement depends on proper surgical technique and patient selection. Distinct surgical considerations exist depending on whether the medial, lateral, or patellofemoral compartment is replaced. Long-term studies have shown that unicompartmental knee replacement is an alternative to total knee arthroplasty.

Marco Kawamura Demange, Marco Sisto, and Scott Rodeo

Arthritis is one of the most frequent musculoskeletal problems, causing pain, disability, and a significant economic burden. In this article, we discuss current nonsurgical injectable treatment options as well as future trends for cartilage lesions and early arthritis of the knee. We cover some potential treatments for knee osteoarthritis, including stem cell and gene therapies.

CLINICS IN SPORTS MEDICINE

Foreword

Unicompartmental Knee Arthritis

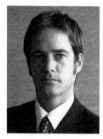 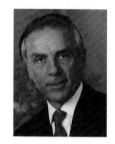

William J. Long, MD, FRCS   W. Norman Scott, MD, FACS

It is our honor and privilege to have this opportunity to address the validity, format, and substance of this symposium.

While at first glance the topic of unicompartmental knee arthritis seems "new," it's not! The American Academy of Orthopedic Surgeons, via the Instructional Course Lectures, addressed this problem, and its application to the younger population in 1993, 20 years ago. The concern at that time was a developing comfort with total knee arthroplasty (TKA) and the application of TKA to both unicompartmental and tricompartmental arthritis, particularly in the younger population. The problem in the 1990s was that the indication for the technology was ill defined due to the sparsity of outcomes for all of the available treatment modalities.

Nonoperative management, medicinal, mechanical, and rehabilitation similarly had limited results on which to indicate certainties of success. As illustrated in this symposium, there is some improvement in the understanding of nonoperative outcomes today and the authors are to be congratulated for illustrating these results.

Biological surgical intervention is unquestionably a seductive approach, but with limited short-term results that must be examined critically; with further experience, we hope to see increased durability. Novel techniques, as mentioned in this symposium, will continue to develop and hopefully be monitored via rigid outcome analysis to allow us to develop appropriate indications.

Currently, as one can surmise from the enclosed articles, the failures of both biological and nonoperative approaches led orthopedists to consider arthroplasty options for the treatment of unicompartmental arthritis, whether it be isolated to the patellofemoral or tibiofemoral compartments. Understanding and applying surgical techniques, such as intramedullary, extramedullary, image-guided, or rapid prototype technology, as discussed in this symposium in great detail, have enhanced the ability to more accurately position unicompartmental implants. Historically, these procedures did not enjoy the same level of reproducibility as total knee procedures, and there was a disparity

Clin Sports Med 33 (2014) xiii–xiv
http://dx.doi.org/10.1016/j.csm.2013.06.007
0278-5919/14/$ – see front matter © 2014 Published by Elsevier Inc.

between individual series and registry results with unicompartmental arthroplasty. Surgeons thus had to consider the reproducibility of the procedure when considering their indications and options. With newer techniques, improved implants and components, reasonable indications, and reproducible surgical techniques, as presented here, unicomparmtental replacement results should continue to improve.

We would like to congratulate Drs Dunn and Plancher for assembling this panel of leaders in the field of unicompartmental arthritis. The topic is timely, well-organized, and critically assessed. The editors and authors should be proud of their accomplishments.

William J. Long, MD, FRCS
Insall Scott Kelly Institute
New York, NY

W. Norman Scott, MD, FACS
Insall Scott Kelly Institute
New York, NY

E-mail addresses:
doctor_long@hotmail.com (W.J. Long)
rosullivan@iskinstitute.com (W.N. Scott)

Note from Consulting Editor

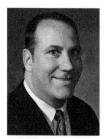

Mark D. Miller, MD
Consulting Editor

My long-time associate and friend, Kevin Plancher, whom I really got to know during our AOSSM traveling fellowship almost two decades ago, has a special interest in unicompartmental knee arthroplasty, and was happy to accept an opportunity to be a guest editor for an issue dedicated to this subject. You may know Dr Plancher as the founder and organizer of the Emerging Technology seminar held the last two years in Las Vegas in December. We were all taken aback by the immediate popularity and success of that course–but if you know Kevin, you really shouldn't be surprised. He has brought the same organizational skills and energy to this issue of Clinics in Sports Medicine–again, no surprise.

The issue begins with non-operative management of unicompartmental knee arthrosis, discusses clinical work-up, and addresses the role of arthroscopy for this condition. ACL instability has long been considered a contraindication to unicompartmental arthroplasty (UKA, or "uni" as it is sometimes referred to), and an entire chapter is devoted to this subject. What follows is a review of several commercially available implants to include robotic assisted UKA's. Chapters on return to activities, outcomes and complications and a look to the future round out this issue. It is a well-organized and well-presented issue, and again we shouldn't be surprised because of the guest editor. Well done, Kevin!

Mark D. Miller, MD
S. Ward Casscells Professor of Orthopaedic Surgery
University of Virginia

Team Physician
James Madison University
JBJS Deputy Editor for Sports Medicine

Director
Miller Review Course
400 Ray C. Hunt Dr, Suite 330
Charlottesville, VA 22908-0159

Clin Sports Med 33 (2014) xv
http://dx.doi.org/10.1016/j.csm.2013.06.008
0278-5919/14/$ – see front matter © 2014 Published by Elsevier Inc.

sportsmed.theclinics.com

Preface

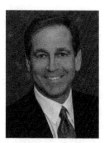

Kevin D. Plancher, MD, MS, FACS, FAAOS
Editor

It is a privilege and honor to serve as editor for this issue of *Clinics in Sports Medicine*. It seems that it was only yesterday when I was asked to edit my first issue of *Clinics in Sports Medicine* 18 years ago. During those years, the increasing recognition of unicompartment arthritis as a treatable disease entity hopefully will make this edition timely for all physicians and surgeons. Perhaps the increasing incidence is due to a better understanding of the anatomy, pathophysiology, clinical symptomatology, and improved surgical techniques.

The early pioneers who treated this disease entity encountered many failures, which encouraged later astute clinicians to forge forward to remedy their errors. Richard Scott, MD, one of my mentors, did just that with his treatise that opened the door for successful outcomes in so many patients, and his article in this issue, "Diagnosis and Indications for Treatment of Unicompartmental Arthritis," hopefully will help all understand his wealth of experience, which has guided us through the years to successfully treat our patients.

The issue's scope traverses the broad spectrum of unicompartmental arthritis. "Nonoperative Treatment of Unicompartmental Arthritis: From Bracing to Injections," written by Jack Bert, MD, teaches us the value of conservative treatment. On the other hand, "Future Trends for Unicompartmental Arthritis of the Knee: Injectables and Stem Cells," written by Scott A. Rodeo, MD, gives us a glimpse of a brilliant clinician and thinker and what is in store in the future or even attempted by some researchers in a limited fashion as he reports on new modalities that search for an intervention for a disease-modifying procedure. Joseph Burkhardt, DO, addresses the role of arthroscopic debridement in "Arthroscopic Debridement of Unicompartmental Arthritis: Fact or Fiction?," a method we have all tried, and brings to light what realistic expectations can be expected. The various prostheses available for unicondylar knee replacement are explored by Anthony Miniaci, MD, with special attention to "UniCAP as an Alternative for Unicompartmental Arthritis." Alan Valadie, MD, shares his experience with a "Unicondylar Knee Arthroplasty: The Arthrex Experience." Aaron Rosenberg, MD, a world-renowned surgeon, shares his success in his article entitled, "The Simple Unicondylar Knee: Extramedullary Technique." I have been asked to contrast this last article with our experience in "Unicondylar Knee Arthroplasty: Intramedullary

Clin Sports Med 33 (2014) xvii–xviii
http://dx.doi.org/10.1016/j.csm.2013.09.001
0278-5919/14/$ – see front matter © 2014 Published by Elsevier Inc.

Technique." This monograph wouldn't be complete without a worldwide experience written by Keith Berend, MD, "Mobile-bearing Unicondylar Knee Arthroplasty: The Oxford Experience." Finally, another glimpse into newer ideas and success is shared by Martin Roche, MD, in "Robotically Assisted Unicondylar Knee Arthroplasty."

While we have come a long way in the development of the unicondylar prosthesis and the technical aspects of surgery for this disease, there is still a need for greater research in this area, particularly around contraindications for unicondylar knee arthroplasty, which we have explored in "The ACL-deficient Knee and Unicompartmental Arthritis," a truly controversial area that I hope will stimulate debate. The last two articles written by veterans in the field, "Outcomes and Complications of Unicondylar Arthroplasty," detailed by Craig Della Valle, MD, and "Patient-Specific Instrumentation and Return to Activities After Unicondylar Knee Arthroplasty," by Joel Boyd, MD, highlight the success of this procedure in returning patients to active lifestyles.

I thank each of the authors, who with their enthusiastic support produced this issue, which I know will guide us all when treating our patients. Special thanks go to Mark Miller, a dear friend, brilliant surgeon, and organizer, who since our first time together has taught me how to expect more of myself, and I am honored to present to him this treatise. Thanks must go to my coeditor, Stephanie Petterson, PhD, a new shining light in the field of orthopedics. Her attention to detail and demands are a role model for all of us. Recognition is noted to Albert Dunn, DO, my fellow, who in beginning his career, has allowed this publication to become print. The culmination of this issue has already shown how important it is to learn what the literature says so we do not repeat the same errors.

DEDICATION

To my mentors, who taught me how to think and to know when to question. To my fellows, who allow me the honor of teaching them. To my colleagues, who give me amazing opportunities. To my mother and father, who encouraged me every day never to give up. To my wife, Jill, my best friend, who understands me better than I understand myself, and last, to my children, Brian, Jamie, and Megan, to whom I ask forgiveness for all those missing moments when I was writing, operating, or seeing patients.

Kevin D. Plancher, MD, MS, FACS, FAAOS
Associate Clinical Professor
Department of Orthopaedics
Albert Einstein College of Medicine
Plancher Orthopaedics and Sports Medicine
1160 Park Avenue
New York, NY 10128, USA

E-mail address:
kplancher@plancherortho.com

Nonoperative Treatment of Unicompartmental Arthritis
From Bracing to Injection

Jack M. Bert, MD[a],*, Timothy M. Bert, MD[b]

KEYWORDS

- Nonoperative treatment • Unicompartmental arthritis • Osteoarthritis • Knee

KEY POINTS

- The primary treatment goals for osteoarthritis (OA) of the knee are to reduce pain, improve joint mobility, and limit functional impairment.
- Pharmacologic treatment options included NSAIDs, COX II inhibitors, and oral non-narcotic analgesics.
- The role of bracing to reduce knee pain in patients with unicompartmental knee OA is helpful to promote a physically active lifestyle and offload the affected joint.
- The use of viscosupplementation for mild to moderate arthritis of the knee and steroid injections for severe arthritis may have value in appropriately selected patients.
- Conservative modalities of the treatment of OA of the knee should be considered before consideration of more aggressive surgical approaches.

INTRODUCTION

The published recommendations for the nonoperative treatment of osteoarthritis (OA) of the knee include weight loss, physical therapy to strengthen lower-extremity musculature, nonsteroidal antiinflammatories, nutritional supplements, topical treatments, and steroid injections. Evidenced-based results have been mixed using these treatment modalities.[1] The results using unloader braces and viscosupplementation have also been variable.[2,3] This article reviews the use of conservative treatment of OA of the knee.

TREATMENT GOALS FOR OA OF THE KNEE

The primary treatment goals for OA of the knee are to reduce pain, improve joint mobility, and limit functional impairment. The secondary goals are to reduce disease

[a] Minnesota Bone & Joint Specialists, Ltd, 17 West Exchange Street, Suite 110, St Paul, MN 55102, USA; [b] Hedley Orthopedic Clinic, 2122 E. Highland Avenue, Suite 300, Phoenix, Arizona
* Corresponding author.
E-mail address: bertx001@umn.edu

Clin Sports Med 33 (2014) 1–10
http://dx.doi.org/10.1016/j.csm.2013.08.002
0278-5919/14/$ – see front matter © 2014 Elsevier Inc. All rights reserved.

progression, improve muscular strength, and, therefore, preserve patients' independence and quality of life.[4] The most effective methods for nonoperatively managing the arthritic knee are behavioral or lifestyle changes. These changes include activity modification, weight loss, and a home therapy and strengthening program. The ultimate goal is to delay joint replacement surgery for as long as possible. Multiple nonpharmacologic treatments have been used, including exercise, weight reduction, thermal modalities, acupuncture, transcutaneous electrical nerve stimulation, shoe insoles and heel wedges, knee braces, and external walking aides, such as canes or walkers.[5]

The Arthritis, Diet, and Activity Promotion Trial was an 18-month-long randomized, single-blinded, clinical trial to determine the impact of exercise and weight loss on the function, pain, and mobility in older overweight and obese adults who had OA of the knee. The investigators found that the combination of modest weight loss plus moderate exercise provided better overall improvements in self-reported measures of function and pain and in performance measures of mobility in older, overweight, and obese adults who had knee OA compared with either intervention alone.[6]

Pharmacologic treatment options include oral analgesics, such as acetaminophen, tramadol, or opioids. Nonsteroidal antiinflammatory drugs (NSAIDs) are the second most commonly prescribe drugs, including ibuprofen (Advil, Motrin) and naproxen (Naprosyn, Aleve). Topical analgesics and patches include diclofenac epolamine (Flector) patches, capsaicin, and lidocaine. Nutraceuticals, such as glucosamine and chondroitin, have also been used. Corticosteroid injections are frequently used for short-term pain relief in patients with significant changes of OA.[7]

The American Geriatric Society considers acetaminophen the initial therapy for mild to moderate musculoskeletal pain, whereas NSAIDs and cyclooxygenase-2 (COX-2) inhibitors, such as celecoxib (Celebrex), are considered secondary therapies. However, some investigators confirmed that acetaminophen is less effective than NSAIDs in relieving OA pain and has no effect on knee stiffness or function in patients with symptomatic knee arthritis.[7,8] An L1 study comparing diclofenac versus acetaminophen, 4000 mg/d, in 82 patients with symptomatic OA of the medial compartment of the knee found acetaminophen to be ineffective.[9] Furthermore, there is a risk of hepatotoxicity, especially if more than 3 g/d are ingested.[10]

Other analgesic medicines include serotonin norepinephrine reuptake inhibitors (SNRIs), such as duloxetine, which are indicated for the management of chronic musculoskeletal pain secondary to chronic OA and chronic lumbar disk disease and spondylosis. SNRIs have been shown to improve pain scores in 2 pivotal trials, but it can result in nausea, fatigue, and constipation and may result in hypertension and abnormal blood sugars in patients with diabetes.[11,12]

Tramadol is useful as a weak opioid agonist and SNRI but runs some risk of abuse. Complications include drowsiness, dizziness, headache, nausea, seizures, and serotonin syndrome. There seems to be less abuse than opioids with respect to drug addiction.[13]

NSAIDs are more effective than acetaminophen for OA pain and are usually the initial treatment modality of OA for orthopedists.[14] NSAIDs reduce pain and inflammation associated with OA by inhibiting the production of prostaglandins in the COX pathway.[15–17] However, usage of NSAIDS results in up to a 30% incidence of peptic ulcers, especially in elderly patients.[18] Furthermore, there is an increase in cardiovascular and cerebrovascular risks and up to 16 500 deaths each year directly or indirectly related to the use of NSAIDS, even in recommended dosages.[18–20] A proton pump inhibitor can be coadministered for higher-risk patients.[7]

The 2 separate COX enzymes that have been described are COX-1 and COX-2. COX-1 enzymes are responsible for producing thromboxane A_2, which involves platelet aggregation, and prostaglandin I_2, which involves gastric mucous production. COX-2 enzymes produce prostaglandin E_2, thought to be the most important inflammatory mediator.[5] The COX-2 drugs preferentially limit inflammation and reduce pain without interfering with the normal production of protective prostaglandins, and thromboxane reduces the incidence of adverse effects. The two separate cyclooxygenase (COX) inhibitor enzymes that have remained in the market and celecoxib and valdecoxib and are significantly more costly than NSAIDs.[21]

Topical analgesics, such as diclofenac gel, patch, or solution, have been recommended as adjunctive or alternative treatments to oral therapy.[7,22] In a prospective randomized trial, pain relief was similar to NSAIDS and side effects were similar to those of placebo.[22]

Capsaicin cream, patch, or solution affects substance P and, although associated with a burning sensation at the site of the patch placement, has a similar mechanism of action and results as diclofenac.[23] Lidocaine patches are used primarily for neuralgia, and the side effects are related to skin rash. Salicylate patches are not recommended for usage in the Osteoarthritis Research Society International's guidelines because of their ineffectiveness.[7]

Glucosamine and chondroitin are commonly used in the treatment of knee OA. A level I study sponsored by the National Institutes of Health with 1583 participants entitled the GAIT study was published in 2006.[24] There was no pain improvement in the overall group but some improvement in the patients with moderate to severe pain. However, a 2010 Cochrane meta-analysis of 3803 patients resulted in no clinically relevant effect on joint pain or radiograph changes. The estimated treatment effects in industry-independent trials were small or absent and clinically irrelevant.[25]

Intraarticular steroid injections are helpful for short-term relief when patients are unresponsive to oral analgesics and NSAIDs or have effusions or synovitis. Furthermore, when patients have significant comorbidities and cannot tolerate oral medication and are unsatisfactory candidates for surgery, intraarticular steroid injections may be indicated every 3 months. Pain relief may last up to 4 weeks.[26] The efficacy of pain relief seems to diminish after 2 years of intraarticular injections performed every 3 months. It seems that the standard of care is to avoid intraarticular injections more frequently than every 3 months.[27,28]

The role of bracing to reduce knee pain in patients with unicompartmental knee OA is helpful to promote a physically active lifestyle and offload the affected joint. This treatment modality is important when considering the effects of contact stress on cartilage and subchondral bone.[29] Knee braces designed to alter joint loading have been developed and modified over the past 30 years and continue to be advocated as a conservative modality for medial or lateral compartment knee OA.[7,30,31] Malalignment of the knee has been shown to increase the progression of medial or lateral compartment OA of the knee.[32] An increase in varus deformity results in an increase in external knee adduction moment (KAM) magnitudes during walking. KAM is associated with a progression in medial knee OA.[33,34] Studies that measure contact stress and joint forces in vivo have reported that a load across the knee joint when walking on a level surface reaches 2 times the body weight (BW) and increases to 3 times the BW when climbing stairs. Jogging at 5 mph increases forces across the knee to 4 times the BW.[35,36]

Using braces to alter loads has been most studied to offload the medial compartment of the knee because the medial compartment is the most common compartment of the knee joint affected with OA.[37] The valgus unloader brace for medial compartment OA is designed to mechanically reorient frontal plane knee alignment to reduce medial tibiofemoral compartment joint loading.[2] Most braces are either prefabricated or custom manufactured and incorporate adjustable straps with thermoplastic cuffs to secure the orthotic to the leg. The braces theoretically provide pain relief by decreasing the load on the medial compartment by applying an opposing external valgus moment about the knee.[35] The improvement in tibiofemoral alignment theoretically shortens the moment arm and reduces KAM, thus unloading the medial compartment.[38] A decrease in muscle cocontraction is the latest theory to explain the benefit of bracing because the offloading effect of bracing has not been shown to be dramatic.[39]

Recent studies have confirmed that there are significant reductions in knee adduction angle measurements[39,40] and in vivo medial loading.[41] Medial compartment joint contact forces have been measured in vivo with 2 valgus braces compared with a non-braced knee. Reductions in medial joint loading were confirmed during walking and stair climbing in test subjects, with a greater reduction when more valgus bracing was performed. The amount of unloading depended on the type of brace, the degree of valgus, and patient tolerance to the external moment applied to the brace.[42] The knee angular impulse and peak KAM were evaluated in a recent simulated study at valgus settings of 4° and 8°. There was a progressive decrease in medial joint loading with increased valgus settings of the brace.[42] Walking distance, gait speed, pain, and muscle strength are all positively influenced by unloader braces.[43–45] Unloader braces have also been shown to improve frontal stability.[39] Younger patients with more severe malalignment and a greater degree of OA may respond more favorably to bracing than older patients with less severe malalignment and a lesser degree of OA.[37,45] Functionally, younger patients tend to do better than older patients[46] and nonobese patients tend to do better with greater pain relief than obese patients.[47] Optimal brace use has, unfortunately, never been defined; however, discomfort from wearing the brace for any significant time has been a deterrent to prolonged brace wear. Poor fit and extremity obesity also contribute to this problem.[41,47] In summary, there is ample recent biomechanical evidence to conclude that valgus bracing reduces load to the medial compartment during walking, stair ascension, and with running activity. However, patient athletic activity and anatomy are significant factors when attempting to determine whether an unloader brace will be helpful in patients with OA.[2]

The usage of viscosupplementation for mild to moderate arthritis of the knee has become increasingly popular in the past 10 to 15 years. Rydell and Balazs[49] first reported the use of intraarticular viscosupplementation injection (IAHA) in dogs in 1971.[48] Before that time, it was used in ophthalmologic surgery.[49] Low-molecular-weight hyaluronan (HA; Hyalgan) was used in Italy in the mid-1980s and Canada in 1992. The Food and Drug Administration (FDA) approved it for use in the United States in 1997 exclusively for the knee. Hyaluronic acid is defined as a device by the FDA[50] and, thus, is regulated as a device in the United States. There are 6 commercially available viscosupplements in the United States at this time: Hyalgan (Sanofi-Synthelabo Inc, Paris, France) has recently been removed from the market after Sanofi purchased Genzyme Corporation in 2012 and now exclusively markets Synvisc, which was approved by the FDA in 1997. Supartz (Seikagaku Corporation, Tokyo, Japan) was released in 2001. Orthovisc (Depuy-Mitek, Inc, Raynham, MA) was released in 2004. Euflexxa (Ferring Pharmaceuticals, Inc, Parsippany, NJ) came to the market in 2004. Gel-One (Zimmer, Inc, Warsaw, IN) was released in 2012. HA is a glycosaminoglycan that consists of N-acetyl-glucosamine and glucuronic acid and is the main component of synovial fluid, and it is found in the cartilage matrix.[49] Type-B synoviocytes, fibroblasts, and chondrocytes synthesize HA, which is secreted into the joint resulting in the viscoelastic properties of hyaluronic acid.[50] The average molecular weight of synovial fluid HA is 4 to 5 $\times$ 10[6] Da.[50–52] In the osteoarthritic joint, the molecular weight decreases by 33% to 50%,[28] which will affect normal joint biomechanics. The mode of action of intraarticular hyaluronic acid results in inhibition of phagocytosis, reduction of prostaglandin synthesis, fibronectin, and clinic adenosine monophosphate levels as well as fibroblastic release of arachidonic acid. Inhibition of nociceptors and decreased synthesis of bradykinin and substance P have been documented with the use of HA.[49,53–56] There are distinct biologic property differences between the compounds that are on the US market. Higher-molecular-weight, cross-linked HA compounds were most effective in stimulating endogenous HA production as well as being chondro-protective when synoviocytes, fibroblasts, and chondrocytes were exposed to interleukin 1, leukocyte proteinases, or oxygen-derived free radicals.[3,57,58] Synvisc and more recently Gel-One are the only 2 cross-linked viscosupplement compounds on the market. Cross-linking occurs when hylan A and hylan B are linked to create a high-molecular-weight compound that has specific actions when injected into the joint. The half-life of cross-linked compounds is 8 to 10 times greater than non–cross-linked compounds, and it is this increase in residence time within the joint that is thought to contribute to greater efficacy with respect to the modes of action of the injected material. However, with cross-linking, there is an increased risk of pseudoseptic reaction that can be reduced by injecting steroids at the same time as administering the injection.[3,59] Analgesic effects can partly be explained HA's antiinflammatory properties and inhibition of nociceptors as well as decreased synthesis of bradykinin and substance P which have been documented with the use of HA.[60,61] The first human clinical trial was published more than 39 years ago when a small group of patients was randomized to IAHA versus placebo and followed over 4 months.[62] Several randomized controlled studies have been published since, and a review of 42 trials from the Agency for Healthcare Research & Quality (AHRQ) report resulted in the American Academy of Orthopaedic Surgeons' (AAOS) clinical practice guidelines (CPG) published in 2009 regarding the treatment of OA of the knee to be inconclusive.[1] However, since then, a Cochrane database review of 76 studies determined that in 5 to 13 weeks status post (S/P) injection, patients treated with IAHA improved in pain, function, and overall assessment.[63,64] In a review of patient series status after arthroscopy for mild to moderate OA of the knee, the usage of viscosupplementation (VS) in these patients has been uniformly successful using visual analog scale (VAS), Western Ontario and McMaster Universities Osteoarthritis Index (WOMAC), and International Knee Documentation Committee (IKDC) scoring systems.[65,66] Postoperative symptomatic improvement has been noted to last from 3.4 months up to 1 year.[67] Several studies have confirmed the benefit of treatment with more than one course of VS. Most patients receiving a second course of therapy have been shown to experience continued pain relief for up to 6 to 12 months after therapy.[68] In another study, Raynaud[69] reported that a second course of therapy with hylan G-F 20 was just as effective as the first course in a study comparing intraarticular HA with conservative care. IAHA may also delay total knee arthroplasty, which may reduce the need for revision surgery, especially in younger patients.[70,71] Using magnetic resonance imaging assessment, cartilage can be preserved in patients with preexisting chondral changes and symptomatic knee OA by receiving IAHA every 6 months over a 2-year period. Tibial volume cartilage was noted to be preserved in the group with OA that had IAHA compared with the control group. The interventional group was also noted to have a reduced annual percentage rate of medial and lateral cartilage tibial volume loss.[72] Animal studies have illustrated that IAHA results in improvement of the quality of regenerated cartilage after microfracture in early time periods after the surgery in rabbits.[73] In a sheep model, IAHA increased the HA concentration and graft articular cartilage quality with a higher concentration of hyaline cartilage proportionate to fibrocartilage.[74] In an anterior cruciate ligament (ACL) reconstruction study using IAHA postoperatively and comparing this group with a saline control, the HA group at 1 year had better functional outcomes and clinical results.[75] The AAOS is currently republishing CPG as well as appropriate use guidelines for usage of IAHA. Unfortunately, the CPG guideline committee only included 14 studies in its analysis and ignored several meta-analyses representing more than 100 studies, including the Cochrane meta-analysis.[63,64,75,76] Of the 14 HA studies included in the AAOS' guideline analysis, 9 studies showed statistical significance with treatment versus placebo. Of those 9 studies, 7 had data to calculate a change or improvement from the baseline, which ranged from 36% to 64%. These mean changes from the baseline exceed the meaningful clinically important improvement (MCII) for meaningful within-patient improvement. Despite this interpretation of the data, the AAOS' CPG guideline committee does not think that there is any indication for the use of IAHA. IAHA is not indicated in patients with complete collapse of the joint space.[76] It has limited indication in the malaligned knee with significant cartilage loss. However, in patients with mild to moderate OA, it seems to be beneficial in halting the progression of OA.[72] Furthermore, using HA in middle-aged patients may result in a delay of total knee arthroplasty and afford patients a more active lifestyle.[70,71] IAHA is a useful treatment modality in patients with OA who are intolerant of NSAIDs. It seems to be helpful after arthroscopy in patients with degenerative changes noted at the time of arthroscopy on the articular surface.[65,66] There seems to be improved results when using higher-molecular-weight HA as opposed to lower-molecular-weight HA because of the increased half-life and residence time within the joint.[77] Further prospective randomized studies in patients with mild to moderate arthritis will be helpful in determining which patients receive the most benefit from this conservative treatment modality.

Conservative modalities of treatment of OA of the knee should be considered before consideration of more aggressive surgical approaches. It is not uncommon to delay surgical intervention by several years by using a home program of weight loss, exercise, pharmacologic treatment, bracing, and injection therapy.

REFERENCES

1. Richmond JR, Hunter D, Irrgang J, et al. AAOS clinical practice guideline summary: treatment of osteoarthritis of the knee (nonarthroplasty). J Am Acad Orthop Surg 2009;17:591–600.
2. Briem K, Ramsey D. The role of bracing. Sports Med Arthrosc 2013;21(1):11–7.
3. Axe J, Snyder-Mackler L, Axe M. The role of viscosupplementation. Sports Med Arthrosc 2013;21(1):18–22.
4. Snibbe JC, Gambardella RA. Orthopedics 2005;28(Suppl 2):215–20.
5. Hanypsiak BT, Shaffer BS. Nonoperative treatment of unicompartmental arthritis of the knee. Orthop Clin North Am 2005;36:401–11.
6. Messier SP, Loeser RF, Miller GD, et al. Exercise and dietary weight loss in overweight and obese older adults with knee osteoarthritis: the Arthritis, Diet, and Activity promotion trial. Arthritis Rheum 2004;50(5):1501–10.
7. Zhang W, Moskowitz R, Nuki G, et al. OARSI recommendations for the management of hip and knee osteoarthritis, part II: OARSI evidence-based, expert consensus guidelines. Osteoarthritis Cartilage 2008;16(2):137–62.
8. Towheed T. Acetaminophen for osteoarthritis. Cochrane Database Syst Rev 2006;(1):CD004257.

9. Case JP, Baliunas AJ, Block JA. Lack of efficacy of acetaminophen in treating symptomatic knee osteoarthritis: a randomized, double-blinded, placebo-controlled comparison trial with diclofenac sodium. Arch Intern Med 2003; 163(2):169–78.

10. Larson L. Acetaminophen-induced acute liver failure: results of a United States multicenter, prospective study. Hepatology 2005;42:1364–72.

11. Chappell C. The use of serotonin uptake inhibitors for chronic pain. Pain Practice 2011;11:1133–41.

12. Chappell C. Duloxetine, a centrally acting analgesic, in the treatment of patients with osteoarthritis knee pain: a 13-week, randomized, placebo-controlled trial. Pain 2009;146:253–60.

13. Nuesch E, et al. Oral or transdermal opioids for osteoarthritis of the knee or hip. Cochrane Database Syst Rev 2009;4:CD003115.

14. Goorman SD, Watanabe TK, Miller EH, et al. Functional outcome in knee osteoarthritis after treatment with hylan G-F 20: a prospective study. Arch Phys Med Rehabil 2008;81:479–83.

15. Bert JM, Gasser SI. Approach to the osteoarthritic knee in the aging athlete: debridement to osteotomy. Arthroscopy 2002;18:107–10.

16. Polisson R. NSAIDs: practical and therapeutic considerations in their selection. Am J Med 1996;100:315–65.

17. Stanley KL, Weaver JE. Pharmacologic management of pain and inflammation in athletes. Clin Sports Med 1998;17:375–92.

18. Rahme E, et al. Hospitalizations for upper and lower GI events associated with traditional NSAIDs and acetaminophen among the elderly in Quebec, Canada. Am J Gastroenterol 2008;103(4):872–82.

19. Barthélémy O, et al. Impact of non-steroidal anti-inflammatory drugs (NSAIDs) on cardiovascular outcomes in patients with stable atherothrombosis or multiple risk factors. Int J Cardiol 2011;163(3):266–71. http://dx.doi.org/10.1016/j.i.jcard.2011.06.015.

20. Abramson SB, Weaver AI. Current state of therapy for pain and inflammation. Arthritis Res Ther 2005;7(Suppl 4):S1–6.

21. Solomon G. The use of COX 2 inhibitors with specific attention to use in patients requiring orthopedic surgical interventions. Orthopedic Special Edition 2002;8: 11–3.

22. Simon LS, et al. Efficacy and safety of topical diclofenac containing dimethyl sulfoxide (DMSO) compared with those of topical placebo, DMSO vehicle and oral diclofenac for knee osteoarthritis. Pain 2009;143:238–45.

23. Altman RD. Practical considerations for the pharmacologic management of osteoarthritis. Am J Manag Care 2009;15(Suppl 8):S236–43.

24. Clegg DO, et al. Glucosamine, chondroitin sulfate, and the two in combination for painful knee osteoarthritis. N Engl J Med 2006;354(8):795–808.

25. Wandel S, et al. Effects of glucosamine, chondroitin, or placebo in patients with osteoarthritis of hip or knee: network meta-analysis. BMJ 2010;341:c4675. http://dx.doi.org/10.1136/bmj.c4675.

26. Bjordal JM, et al. Short-term efficacy of pharmacotherapeutic interventions in osteoarthritic knee pain: a meta-analysis of randomised placebo-controlled trials. Eur J Pain 2007;11:125–38.

27. Raynaud JP, et al. Safety and efficacy of long-term intraarticular steroid injections in osteoarthritis of the knee: a randomized, double-blind, placebo-controlled trial. Arthritis Rheum 2003;48:370–7.

28. Dahmer S, Schiller RM. Glucosamine. Am Fam Physician 2008;78(4):471–6, 481.

29. Vignon E, Valat JP, Rossignol M, et al. Osteoarthritis of the knee and hip and activity: a systematic international review and synthesis (OASIS). Joint Bone Spine 2006;73:442–55.
30. Pollo F, Jackson R. Knee bracing for unicompartmental osteoarthritis. J Am Acad Orthop Surg 2006;14:5–11.
31. Ramsey D, Russell M. Unloader braces for knee braces for knee osteoarthritis: implications on preventing progression. Sports Health 2009;1:416–26.
32. Sharma L, Song J, Felson D, et al. The role of knee alignment in disease progression and functional decline in knee osteoarthritis. JAMA 2001;286: 188–95.
33. Miyazaki T, Wada M, Kawahara H, et al. Dynamic load at baseline can predict radiographic disease progression in medial compartment knee osteoarthritis. Ann Rheum Dis 2002;61:617–22.
34. Hurwitz D, Ryals A, Case J, et al. The knee adduction moment during gait in subjects with knee osteoarthritis is more closely correlated with static alignment than radiographic disease severity, toe out angle and pain. J Orthop Res 2002; 20:101–7.
35. Kutzner I, Heinlein B, Graichen F, et al. Loading of the knee joint during activities of daily living measured in vivo in five subjects. J Biomech 2010;43:2164–73.
36. D'Lima D, Steklov N, Patil S, et al. The Mark Coventry Award: in vivo knee forces during recreation and exercise after knee arthroplasty. Clin Orthop Relat Res 2008;466:2605–11.
37. Pollo F, Otis J, Backus S, et al. Reduction of medial compartment loads with valgus bracing of the osteoarthritic knee. Am J Sports Med 2002;30:414–21.
38. Gross K, Hillstrom H. Noninvasive devices targeting the mechanics of osteoarthritis. Rheum Dis Clin North Am 2008;34:755–76.
39. Ramsey D, Briem K, Axe M, et al. A mechanical theory for the effectiveness of bracing for medial compartment osteoarthritis of the knee. J Bone Joint Surg Am 2007;89:2398–3407.
40. Draganich L, Reider B, Rimington T. The effectiveness of self-adjustable custom and off – the –shelf bracing in the treatment of varus gonarthrosis. J Bone Joint Surg Am 2006;88:2645–52.
41. Kutzner I, Kuther S, Heinlein B, et al. The effect of valgus braces on medial compartment load of the knee joint-in vivo load measurements in three subjects. J Biomech 2011;44:1354–60.
42. Fantini Pagani C, Hinrichs M, Bruggemann G. Kinetic and kinematic changes with the use of valgus knee brace and lateral wedge insoles in patients with medial knee osteoarthritis. J Orthop Res 2012;30:1125–32.
43. Gaasbeek R, Groen B, Hampsink B, et al. Valgus bracing in patients with medial compartment osteoarthritis of the knee: a gait analysis study of a new brace. Gait Posture 2007;26:3–10.
44. Schmalz T, Knopf E, Drewitz H, et al. Analysis of biomechanical effectiveness of valgus-inducing knee brace for osteoarthritis of knee. J Rehabil Res Dev 2010; 47:419–29.
45. Brouwer R, van Raaij T, Verhaar H, et al. Brace treatment of osteoarthritis of the knee: a prospective randomized mutli-centre trial. Osteoarthritis Cartilage 2006; 14:777–83.
46. Hewett T, Noyes F, Barber-Westin S, et al. Decrease in knee joint pain and increase in function in patients with medial compartment arthrosis: a prospective analysis of valgus bracing. Orthopedics 1998;21:131–8.

47. Dennis A, Komistek R. An in vivo analysis of the effectiveness of the osteoarthritic knee brace during heel strike and midstance of gait. Acta Chir Orthop Traumatol Cech 1999;66:323–7.
48. Rydell N, Balazs E. Effect of intra-articular injection of hyaluronic acid on the clinical symptoms of osteoarthritis and on granulation tissue formation. Clin Orthop 1971;80:25–32.
49. Balazs E, Denlinger J. Viscosupplementation: a new concept in the treatment of osteoarthritis. J Rheumatol Suppl 1993;39:3–9.
50. Brockmeier S, Shaffer B. Viscosupplementation therapy for osteoarthritis. Sports Med Arthrosc 2006;14:155–62.
51. Conduah A, Baker C. Managing joint pain in osteoarthritis: safety and efficacy of hylan G-F 20. J Pain Res 2009;2:87–98.
52. Watterson J, Esdaile J. Viscosupplementation: therapeutic mechanisms and clinical potential in osteoarthritis of the knee. J Am Acad Orthop Surg 2000;8:277–84.
53. Forrester J, Balazs E. Inhibition of phagocytosis by high molecular weight hyaluronate. Immunology 1980;40:435–46.
54. Hakansson L, Hallegran R, Venge P. Regulation of granulocyte function by hyaluronic acid: in vitro and in vivo effects on phagocytosis, locomotion and metabolism. J Clin Invest 1980;66:298–305.
55. Balazs EA, Watson D, Duff IF, et al. Hyaluronic acid in synovial fluid: I. Molecular parameters of hyaluronic acid in normal and arthritis human fluids. Arthritis Rheum 1967;10:357–76.
56. Felson D, Lawrence R, Dieppe P, et al. Osteoarthritis: new insights. Part 1: the disease and its risk factors. Ann Intern Med 2000;133:635–46.
57. Smith M, Ghosh P. The synthesis of hyaluronic acid by human synovial fibroblasts is influenced by the nature of the hyaluronate in the extracellular environment. Rheumatol Int 1987;7:113–22.
58. Ghosh P. The role of hyaluronic acid (hyaluronan) in health and disease: interactions with cells, cartilage and components of synovial fluid. Clin Exp Rheumatol 1994;12:75–82.
59. Leopold S, Warme W, Pettis P, et al. Increased frequency of acute local reaction to intra-articular hylan GF-20 (Synvisc) in patients receiving more than one course of treatment. J Bone Joint Surg Am 2002;84:1619–23.
60. Moreland L. Intra-articular hyaluronan (hyaluronic acid) and hylans for the treatment of osteoarthritis: mechanisms of action. Arthritis Res Ther 2003;5:54–67.
61. Gomis A, Pawlak M, Balazs E, et al. Effects of different molecular weight elastoviscous hyaluronan solutions on articular nociceptive afferents. Arthritis Rheum 2004;50:314–26.
62. Peyron J, Balasz E. Preliminary clinical assessment of Na-hyaluronate injection into human arthritic joints. Pathol Biol (Paris) 1974;22:731–6.
63. Bellamy N, Campbell J, Robinson V, et al. Viscosupplementation for the treatment of osteoarthritis of the knee. Cochrane Database Syst Rev 2006;(2):CD005321.
64. Bellamy N, Campbell J, Robinson V, et al. Viscosupplementation for the treatment of osteoarthritis of the knee. Cochrane Database Syst Rev 2006;(2):CD005328.
65. Bert J, Waddell D. Viscosupplementation with hylan G-F 20 in patients with osteoarthrosis of the knee. Ther Adv Musculoskel Dis 2010;2(3):127–32.
66. Waddell D, Bert J. The use of hyaluronan after arthroscopic surgery of the knee. Arthroscopy 2010;26(1):105–11.

67. Hempfling H. Intra-articular hyaluronic acid after knee arthroscopy: a two-year study. Knee Surg Sports Traumatol Arthrosc 2010;15:537–46.

68. Waddell D, Cefalu C, Bricker D. A second course of hylan G-F 20 for the treatment of osteoarthritic knee pain: 12 month follow-up. J Knee Surg 2005;18(1): 7–15.

69. Raynaud J. Effectiveness and safety of repeat courses of hylan G-F 20 in patients with knee osteoarthritis. Osteoarthritis Cartilage 2005;13:111–9.

70. Burns W, Bourne R, Chesworth B, et al. Cost effectiveness of revision total knee arthroplasty. Clin Orthop Relat Res 2006;446:29–33.

71. Waddell D, Bricker D. Total knee replacement delayed with hylan G-F 20 use in patients with grade IV osteoarthritis. J Manag Care Pharm 2007;13:113–21.

72. Wang Y, Hall S, Hanna F, et al. Effects of hylan G-F 20 supplementation on cartilage preservation detected by magnetic resonance imaging in osteoarthritis of the knee: a two year single-blind clinical trial. BMC Musculoskelet Disord 2011; 12:195–203.

73. Strauss E, Schachter A, Frenkel S, et al. The efficacy of intra-articular hyaluronan injection after microfracture technique for the treatment of articular cartilage lesions. Am J Sports Med 2009;37:720–6.

74. Tytherleigh-Strong G, Hurtig M, Miniaci A. Intra-articular hyaluron following autogenous osteochondral grafting of the knee. Arthroscopy 2005;21:999–1005.

75. Bannuru RR, Natov NS, Obadan IE, et al. Therapeutic trajectory of hyaluronic acid versus corticosteroids in the treatment of knee osteoarthritis: a systematic review and meta-analysis. Arthritis Rheum 2009;61:1704–11.

76. Wang C, Lin J, Chang C, et al. Therapeutic effects of hyaluronic acid on osteoarthritis of the knee. A meta-analysis of randomized controlled trials. J Bone Joint Surg Am 2004;86:538–45.

77. Zhang W, Nuki G, Moskowitz RW, et al. OARSI recommendations for the management of hip and knee osteoarthritis: part III. Changes in evidence following systematic cumulative update of research published through January 2009. Osteoarthritis Cartilage 2010;18:476–99.

Diagnosis and Indications for Treatment of Unicompartmental Arthritis

Brian T. Palumbo, MD[a],*, Richard D. Scott, MD[b]

KEYWORDS

- Unicompartmental knee arthroplasty • Arthritis • Knee • Diagnosis and indications

KEY POINTS

- Unicompartmental knee arthroplasty continues to be an evolving procedure with highly specific indications that are closely associated with clinical outcome and survivorship.
- As surgical techniques and implant designs improve, the indications for UKA will probably continue to expand and their successes improve.
- Technical experience and a comprehensive understanding of patient factors such as age, activity level and patient weight can dramatically impact long-term results and should guide treatment.
- The senior author warns of potentially lower long-term survivorship in the young, active mesomorphic male patient.
- Medial compartment osteoarthritis that leads to attritional rupture of the ACL is frequently too advanced for successful UKA. However, acute or subacute ACL rupture with early posterior-medial compartment wear can be successfully treated with concomitant UKA/ACL reconstruction.

INTRODUCTION

Advances in surgical technique and implant design have improved clinical outcomes and survivorship in total knee arthroplasty (TKA). This improvement, however, cannot be said to the same extent for unicompartmental knee arthroplasty (UKA) (Fig. 1).[1] Despite significant functional advantages of UKA compared with TKA under the appropriate circumstances,[2–5] indications for UKA remain stringent, and advances in clinical outcome and survivorship continue to be limited.[1,6–9]

UKA's prolonged development is partially related to the relative infrequency of performance of UKA versus TKA. Other reasons include implant design[10–12] and technical considerations that directly impact implant longevity.[13–15] Although some authors report good long-term survivorship, other series, such as European registry data,

[a] Harvard Combined Orthopaedics, Brigham and Women's Hospital, 75 Francis Street, Boston, MA 02115, USA; [b] Harvard Medical School, 125 Parker Hill Avenue, Suite 560, Boston, MA 02120, USA
* Corresponding author.
E-mail address: bpalumbo79@gmail.com

Clin Sports Med 33 (2014) 11–21
http://dx.doi.org/10.1016/j.csm.2013.06.001
0278-5919/14/$ – see front matter © 2014 Elsevier Inc. All rights reserved.

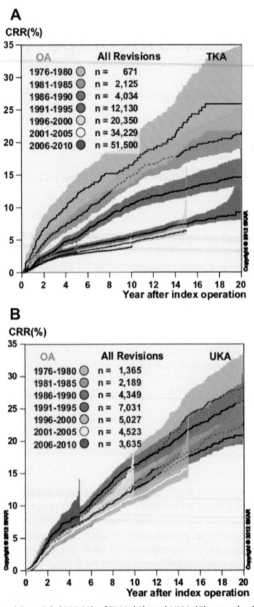

Fig. 1. Cumulative revision risk (CRR%) of TKA (*A*) and UKA (*B*) over the last several decades. Over time, TKA survivorship has improved dramatically, whereas UKA has not experienced the same advances in longevity. (*From* the 2012 Swedish Knee Arthroplasty Registry Annual Report; with permission.)

report inferior results.[1,6–8] A comprehensive understanding of these issues and their relationship to patient selection, diagnosis, and management is crucial for maximizing successful long-term results.

Achieving acceptable long-term outcomes and survivorship can be more challenging than TKA. Consequences of slight malposition and knee imbalance are more detrimental because of patient factors and technical reasons specific to UKA candidates. Malalignment of as little as 3° and just 3 mm of tibial overhang have each been shown to increase strain at the tibial baseplate bone-cement interface by as much as 40% in finite element analyses.[15] Implant design, especially relating to the baseplate and fixation, plays an integral biomechanical role in countering the ill effects of malalignment and diminishes the potential for baseplate loosening. Additionally, although traditional criteria limit UKA to low-demand patients,[16] there has been an expansion of indications to treat younger or higher-demand patients who would benefit from the functional advantages of retained cruciate ligaments and improved proprioception that UKA offers. Unfortunately, these patients impart greater stress on UKA components which can expedite component loosening. Furthermore, clinical factors such as high body weight and anterior cruciate ligament (ACL) incompetence result in greater implant loading and altered knee kinematics, further threatening the life of the implant. A comprehensive understanding of all of these factors is crucial to obtain reproducibly good initial clinical results and long-term survivability.

INDICATIONS AND PATIENT SELECTION

The stringent criteria published by Kozinn and colleagues[17] in 1989 have maintained certain relevance over the last several decades. The criteria consist of the following: isolated medial or lateral compartment arthritis or osteonecrosis, low-demand activity with weight less than 82 kg (181 lbs), and age greater than 60 years. The patient should have minimal pain at rest, range of motion arc greater than 90° with less than 5° flexion contracture, and an angular deformity of less than 15° that is passively correctable.

Their proposed *contraindications* to UKA were the following:

• Diagnosis of inflammatory arthritis
• Patient age less than 60 years
• High patient activity level
• Pain at rest (which could indicate an inflammatory component to the arthropathy)
• Patellofemoral pain
• Exposed bone in the patellofemoral joint or opposite compartment

Although excellent results have been reported with application of these guidelines,[18] their stringency limits the applicability of UKA to a relatively small population of low-demand patients. Ritter and colleagues[19] reported that of 4021 cases of knee arthritis, only 6.1% of patients met the anatomic/radiographic criteria, and 4.3% met the clinical criteria. Stern and colleagues[20] also estimated a similarly low percentage of patients. Although the stringent standards of Kozinn and Scott serve to improve the likelihood of clinical success and survivorship, it also means that the procedure will rarely be performed by any but the experienced arthroplasty surgeon. Furthermore, it limits the operation to patients who are less likely to benefit from the functional and proprioceptive advantages of UKA. In elderly low-demand patients, TKA provides a reliable means for improved function and pain relief with better survival than UKA in most studies.[1,7] Despite these limitations, however, over the last several decades, surgeons have expanded UKA criteria in an attempt to apply the functional and bone-preserving benefits of UKA to younger and more active patients.

UKA in the Young

The application of UKA to younger, higher-demand patients has been met with mixed results. Swienckowski and Pennington[21] reported 92% survivorship at a mean follow-up of 11 years in 45 UKA patients younger than 60 years. In surviving patients he reported 100% good or excellent results and a mean postoperative alignment of 5° valgus. Felts and colleagues[22] reported 94% survivorship at 12 years in 65 patients younger than 60 years. Additionally, they observed significant improvement in knee society scores, and 83.4% of patients returned to sporting activities. Similar results of good clinical outcomes and survivorship can be found throughout the literature. However, many of these publications are generated from surgeons and institutions that perform large numbers of knee arthroplasties, specifically, UKAs. These data skew the perception that UKA can be performed in young, active patients with reproducibly good results and long-term survivorship. This notion is sharply contrasted by European and Australian knee arthroplasty registries that consistently show poorer clinical results and higher revision rates in patients younger than 65 years.[1,6–8] The heterogeneous nature of registry data consisting of varying surgeon experience and technical ability as well as different implant designs may be more applicable to the general orthopedic community than experienced, high-volume surgeons or centers. Although age and activity level most certainly influence outcome and survivorship in UKA, its negative impact is countered by the surgeon's expertise. Current UKA implants are intolerant of malalignment; therefore, accurate and precise implantation is paramount to achieving reproducibly good results in the young. Although these issues should be in the forefront when considering UKA in a young, active individual, they should not exclude a patient who might benefit from UKA either. Proceeding with a TKA for symptomatic unicompartmental disease in a young patient simply because other nonarthroplasty options lack promise has inherent flaws. Although TKA may provide reliable pain relief, function is inferior to that of UKA, and patients are committed to a more complex revision in the future. Relative to alternatives such as medical management, osteotomy, and TKA, UKA may be the best option in providing reliable pain relief and optimal function with limited morbidity. Later conversion to TKA can be accomplished successfully, sometimes necessitating revision components such as stems or augments or bone graft.[23,24] A conservative initial tibial resection during UKA has been shown to be key for successful conversion to TKA using primary components.[25] Good long-term clinical success can be achieved with conversion to TKA, although some report inferior outcomes compared with TKA in the primary setting.[7,26,27]

Although a perfect surgical solution for this patient population remains elusive, a reliable approach is one that accounts for individual patient characteristics and needs. Additionally, a comprehensive understanding of expectations and limitations of UKA in the young patient is necessary of the surgeon and patient.

UKA in the Obese

Obesity adds an additional level of complexity in UKA and lacks a consensus in the literature. The obese patient typically presents earlier because of excessive tibiofemoral loads and premature compartment degeneration. Patients often are not only obese but also young, further complicating the treatment decision. Excess weight translates to greater implant interface stress and increases the potential for early implant loosening, especially in the setting of component malposition. Mont and colleagues compared 40 fixed-bearing UKA patients with a body mass index (BMI) less than 35 and 40 cases with those with a BMI greater than 35. He observed an increased revision rate and poorer knee society scores in obese patients.[28] Berend and colleagues[29] evaluated 79 UKAs with a mean follow-up of 40 months and observed that a BMI greater than 32 was an independent risk factor for implant failure and diminished survivorship. In this series, two variations of cemented all-polyethylene tibial components were used. This design lacks a tibial keel and the added stability it affords. Component fixation is crucial in higher-weight patients and may have impacted the results of this study. Contrary results of success with UKA in higher-weight patients have been reported as well. Kuipers and colleagues[30] studied 437 Oxford III UKAs and observed a greater than 2-fold risk of revision in patients younger than 60 years. They did not, however, find that a BMI greater than 30 affected clinical outcome or implant survivorship. In a study by Xing and colleagues,[31] of 178 UKAs and a mean follow-up of 54 months, obesity was not found to be a risk factor for failure. In the senior author's experience, it is the active middle-age mesomorphic male patient, not the obese female, who presents the highest risk for eventual femoral or tibial component loosening.

UKA in the ACL-Deficient Knee

Utility of UKA in the ACL-deficient knee has expanded over the last several decades. One of 2 distinct clinical scenarios can exist. An understanding of these differing pathogeneses of concomitant unicompartmental arthritis and ACL deficiency can help direct surgical planning and avoid poor outcomes. A differentiation should be made between "ACL deficiency caused by unicompartmental arthritis" and "unicompartmental arthritis caused by an ACL deficiency." Primary unicompartmental arthritis begins at the anteromedial aspect of the knee and advances posteriorly to involve the femoral condyle and intercondylar notch. Inflammation elicited by cartilage degradation and ACL impingement by femoral notch osteophytes creates a biochemical and mechanical milieu for ACL destruction.[32,33] Once ACL disruption has occurred, knee kinematics worsen, further exacerbating posterior-medial compartment degeneration. The medial collateral ligament (MCL) eventually shortens and contracts, furthering the advancement of the degenerative process to the lateral compartment. UKA may be an early option during this process and may, theoretically, slow the progression of disease to the contralateral compartment if normal kinematics can be approximated. This finding is supported by McCallum and Scott[34] who found that a preoperative anterior-medial wear pattern frequently results in a similar polyethylene wear pattern after UKA. This wear pattern is best seen preoperatively in a lateral x-ray taken with the knee in extension. In their study, they theorized that the medial compartment is subjected to similar stress after UKA.

After attritional ACL disruption occurs, the wear pattern will continue to the posterior third of the medial compartment. A UKA is not advisable in these circumstances and has been fraught with poor results.[35,36] Goodfellow and O'Connor[35] reported a 95% and 81% survivorship with mobile bearing UKAs at 6 years in ACL intact and deficient knees, respectively. Increased roll back results in posteriorized contact loading and a rocking phenomenon of the baseplate to occur, leading to increased strain at the anterior tibial bone-cement interface.[36–38] The small baseplate surface area and cement fixation resist strain poorly, leading to implant-interface pain and loosening. This effect may be limited by decreasing tibial slope as shown by Hernigou and Deschamps.[39] They observed improved survivorship in ACL-deficient knees when the tibial slope was less than 7°.

Lateral Compartment UKA and ACL Deficiency

The aforementioned difficulties are amplified in the setting of lateral unicompartmental disease. In the native knee, lateral compartment motion is substantially greater than that of the medial compartment and is exaggerated with ACL incompetence. Abnormal kinematics and the subsequent deleterious stresses on UKA components are only exacerbated in the lateral compartment with ACL incompetence and therefore is contraindicated.[40]

Concomitant UKA and ACL Reconstruction

When the initiating event in unicompartmental arthritis is ACL disruption, the pattern of joint degeneration as well as treatment options differ. ACL disruption in the native knee leads to increased tibial subluxation and translation, resulting in excessive shear in the posterior-medial compartment. This shear results in attritional meniscal and cartilage damage and posterior medial compartment arthritis.[41] This degenerative pattern is evident on PA radiographs with the knee in a 30° flexed position. With the knee flexed and no ACL to prevent excess anterior tibial translation, the medial femoral condyle translates into the posterior-medial tibial defect, and the true severity of the joint degeneration can be visualized radiographically. These patients are typically younger and more active with intact collateral ligaments and preserved lateral and patellofemoral compartments. Either staged or simultaneous UKA and ACL reconstruction has emerged as a viable option for this circumstance.

Weston-Simons and colleagues[42] reported a 93% survivorship and satisfaction in all but one patient in 52 simultaneous or staged UKA with ACL reconstructions. In this series, the decision to proceed with a simultaneous or staged UKA/ACL reconstruction was dependent on whether the patient's main complaint was instability (staged with ACL first) or instability with pain (simultaneous reconstruction). Tinius and colleagues[43] reported significant improvements in knee society scores, no recurrence of instability, and a 100% survivorship in 27 patients after combined UKA/ACL reconstruction at 53 months. Kinematic studies corroborate the clinical results supporting combined UKA/ACL reconstruction.[44,45] Pandit and colleagues[44] analyzed step-up exercises and deep knee bends with fluoroscopy in 10 Oxford UKA patients, 10 Oxford UKA/ACL reconstruction patients, and 22 native knee patients. Similar knee kinematics was observed in all 3 groups, and similar mobile bearing movement was observed in the UKA and UKA/ACL specimens.

UKA in the Setting of Patellofemoral Arthritis

Although UKA in the setting of patellofemoral arthritis (PFA) was previously considered a contraindication, this notion has been successfully contested in most recent studies. Although some continue to maintain that at least symptomatic PFA should be a contraindication, other authors simply and successfully ignore its presence. Beard and colleagues[46] prospectively analyzed 824 consecutive mobile-bearing Oxford UKA patients for the presence of intraoperative full-thickness cartilage loss. They concluded that the severity of patellofemoral cartilage loss had no impact on outcome and should not be considered a contraindication to Oxford UKA as long as lateral facet grooving or bone loss was nonexistent. Beard and others[47] also analyzed the impact of preoperative patellofemoral symptoms and radiographic evidence of PFA on clinical outcomes 2 years postoperatively. Preoperatively, 54% of patients had patellofemoral pain and 54% had radiographic PFA but were found to have similar clinical outcomes to those without PFA. Price and colleagues,[48] who ignored the preoperative state of the patellofemoral joint, reported no failures for patellofemoral complications in 114 mobile-bearing UKA patients at 10 years. Additionally, 97% of patients lacked patellofemoral pain at final follow-up.

Combined UKA and Patellofemoral Arthroplasty

Combined patellofemoral and tibiofemoral unicompartmental arthroplasty has emerged as an alternative to ignoring the patellofemoral joint. Options consist of individualized resurfacing of each of these compartments or use of monoblock femoral components that resurfaces the patellofemoral and affected tibiofemoral joints. The

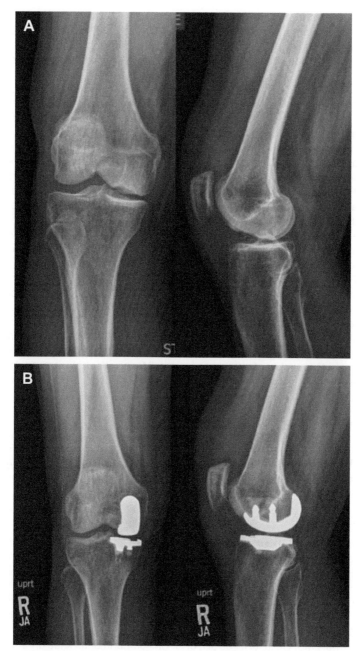

Fig. 2. (*A*) Preoperative anteroposterior and lateral radiograph of a 68-year-old woman with isolated osteonecrosis of the medial femoral condyle. (*B*) Postoperative radiographs after successful medial unicompartmental arthroplasty.

success of bicompartmental arthroplasty is inconclusive to date with relatively few and small clinical studies supporting this technique. Although early results of individualized compartment resurfacing is promising,[49] resurfacing dual compartments with mono-block femoral components was met with unacceptable outcomes in one study.[50]

UKA in the Setting of Osteonecrosis

For UKA in the setting of osteonecrosis, differentiation between primary and secondary disease is crucial, as the literature is disparate regarding these 2 pathologies.[51–53] Primary osteonecrosis typically affects patients older than 55 years, impacts a single compartment, and is unilateral. Secondary osteonecrosis can be elicited by corticosteroid use, alcoholism, chronic renal failure, and barotrauma. Additionally, involvement of multiple compartments and multiple joints is frequent with secondary osteonecrosis. Bruni and colleagues[51] reviewed 84 UKA patients for late-stage, spontaneous osteonecrosis and reported an 89% 10-year survivorship. The most common cause for revision in this series was tibial component subsidence. All cases of secondary osteonecrosis were excluded in this study, however. Heyse and colleagues[52] reported 97% satisfaction and 90% survival at 15 years in 52 UKAs for spontaneous osteonecrosis of the knee. While these studies considered secondary osteonecrosis a contraindication, Parratte and colleagues[53] reviewed 31 UKAs for the treatment of both primary and secondary osteonecrosis. This series consisted of 21 primary and 10 secondary osteonecrosis cases. Patient selection criteria consisted of osteonecrosis involvement of a single femoral condyle, fully correctable deformity on stress radiographs, preserved patellofemoral joint, and a competent ACL. Although excellent functional results and a survival rate of 97% at 12 years were obtained in both primary and secondary osteonecrosis, the number of cases was too small for an adequate statistical comparison of the 2 groups. In our experience, as long as the osteonecrotic involvement is not extensive, excellent outcomes can be expected in most cases (**Fig. 2**).

SUMMARY

UKA offers definite advantages in function, proprioception and bone preservation compared to TKA. A comprehensive understanding of patient factors, knee pathology and implant design may help guide surgical management and impact clinical outcomes and survivorship.

REFERENCES

1. Department of Orthopaedics SUHL. Swedish Knee Arthroplasty Register. 2012.
2. Rougraff BT, Heck DA, Gibson AE. A comparison of tricompartmental and unicompartmental arthroplasty for the treatment of gonarthrosis. Clin Orthop Relat Res 1991;(273):157–64.
3. Laurencin CT, Zelicof SB, Scott RD, et al. Unicompartmental versus total knee arthroplasty in the same patient. A comparative study. Clin Orthop Relat Res 1991;(273):151–6.
4. Noticewala MS, Geller JA, Lee JH, et al. Unicompartmental knee arthroplasty relieves pain and improves function more than total knee arthroplasty. J Arthroplasty 2012;27(Suppl 8):99–105.
5. Sun PF, Jia YH. Mobile bearing UKA compared to fixed bearing TKA: a randomized prospective study. Knee 2012;19(2):103–6.
6. Baker PN, Petheram T, Avery PJ, et al. Revision for unexplained pain following unicompartmental and total knee replacement. J Bone Joint Surg Am 2012; 94(17):e126.

7. Pearse AJ, Hooper GJ, Rothwell A, et al. Survival and functional outcome after revision of a unicompartmental to a total knee replacement: the New Zealand National Joint Registry. J Bone Joint Surg Br 2010;92(4):508–12.
8. W-Dahl A, Robertsson O, Lidgren L, et al. Unicompartmental knee arthroplasty in patients aged less than 65. Acta Orthop 2010;81(1):90–4.
9. Koskinen E, Paavolainen P, Eskelinen A, et al. Unicondylar knee replacement for primary osteoarthritis: a prospective follow-up study of 1,819 patients from the Finnish Arthroplasty Register. Acta Orthop 2007;78(1):128–35.
10. Walker PS, Parakh DS, Chaudhary ME, et al. Comparison of interface stresses and strains for onlay and inlay unicompartmental tibial components. J Knee Surg 2011;24(2):109–15.
11. Small SR, Berend ME, Ritter MA, et al. Metal backing significantly decreases tibial strains in a medial unicompartmental knee arthroplasty model. J Arthroplasty 2011;26(5):777–82.
12. Small SR, Berend ME, Ritter MA, et al. Bearing mobility affects tibial strain in mobile-bearing unicompartmental knee arthroplasty. Surg Technol Int 2010;19:185–90.
13. Chau R, Gulati A, Pandit H, et al. Tibial component overhang following unicompartmental knee replacement–does it matter? Knee 2009;16(5):310–3.
14. Iesaka K, Tsumura H, Sonoda H, et al. The effects of tibial component inclination on bone stress after unicompartmental knee arthroplasty. J Biomech 2002;35(7):969–74.
15. Simpson DJ, Price AJ, Gulati A, et al. Elevated proximal tibial strains following unicompartmental knee replacement–a possible cause of pain. Med Eng Phys 2009;31(7):752–7.
16. Kozinn S, Scott R. Unicondylar knee arthroplasty. J Bone Joint Surg Am 1989;71(1):145–50.
17. Kozinn SC, Marx C, Scott RD. Unicompartmental knee arthroplasty. A 4.5-6-year follow-up study with a metal-backed tibial component. J Arthroplasty 1989;(Suppl 4):S1–10.
18. Berger RA, Meneghini RM, Jacobs JJ, et al. Results of unicompartmental knee arthroplasty at a minimum of ten years of follow-up. J Bone Joint Surg Am 2005;87(5):999–1006.
19. Ritter MA, Faris PM, Thong AE, et al. Intra-operative findings in varus osteoarthritis of the knee. An analysis of pre-operative alignment in potential candidates for unicompartmental arthroplasty. J Bone Joint Surg Br 2004;86(1):43–7.
20. Stern SH, Becker MW, Insall JN. Unicondylar knee arthroplasty. An evaluation of selection criteria. Clin Orthop Relat Res 1993;(286):143–8.
21. Swienckowski JJ, Pennington DW. Unicompartmental knee arthroplasty in patients sixty years of age or younger. J Bone Joint Surg Am 2004;86-A(Suppl 1(Pt 2)):131–42.
22. Felts E, Parratte S, Pauly V, et al. Function and quality of life following medial unicompartmental knee arthroplasty in patients 60 years of age or younger. Orthop Traumatol Surg Res 2010;96(8):861–7.
23. Levine WN, Ozuna RM, Scott RD, et al. Conversion of failed modern unicompartmental arthroplasty to total knee arthroplasty. J Arthroplasty 1996;11(7):797–801.
24. Springer BD, Scott RD, Thornhill TS. Conversion of failed unicompartmental knee arthroplasty to TKA. Clin Orthop Relat Res 2006;446:214–20.
25. Schwarzkopf R, Mikhael B, Li L, et al. Revision of medial unicompartmental arthroplasty of the knee: does initial tibial resection thickness affect outcome of revision. J Orthop 2013;36(4):e409–14.

26. Chou DT, Swamy GN, Lewis JR, et al. Revision of failed unicompartmental knee replacement to total knee replacement. Knee 2012;19(4):356–9.

27. Rancourt MF, Kemp KA, Plamondon SM, et al. Unicompartmental knee arthroplasties revised to total knee arthroplasties compared with primary total knee arthroplasties. J Arthroplasty 2012;27(Suppl 8):106–10.

28. Bonutti PM, Goddard MS, Zywiel MG, et al. Outcomes of unicompartmental knee arthroplasty stratified by body mass index. J Arthroplasty 2011;26(8):1149–53.

29. Berend KR, Lombardi AV Jr, Mallory TH, et al. Early failure of minimally invasive unicompartmental knee arthroplasty is associated with obesity. Clin Orthop Relat Res 2005;440:60–6.

30. Kuipers BM, Kollen BJ, Bots PC, et al. Factors associated with reduced early survival in the Oxford phase III medial unicompartment knee replacement. Knee 2010;17(1):48–52.

31. Xing Z, Katz J, Jiranek W. Unicompartmental knee arthroplasty: factors influencing the outcome. J Knee Surg 2012;25(5):369–74.

32. White SH, Ludkowski PF, Goodfellow JW. Anteromedial osteoarthritis of the knee. J Bone Joint Surg Br 1991;73(4):582–6.

33. Hasegawa A, Otsuki S, Pauli C, et al. Anterior cruciate ligament changes in the human knee joint in aging and osteoarthritis. Arthritis Rheum 2012;64(3):696–704.

34. McCallum JD 3rd, Scott RD. Duplication of medial erosion in unicompartmental knee arthroplasties. J Bone Joint Surg Br 1995;77(5):726–8.

35. Goodfellow J, O'Connor J. The anterior cruciate ligament in knee arthroplasty. A risk-factor with unconstrained meniscal prostheses. Clin Orthop Relat Res 1992;(276):245–52.

36. Goodfellow JW, Kershaw CJ, Benson MK, et al. The Oxford Knee for unicompartmental osteoarthritis. The first 103 cases. J Bone Joint Surg Br 1988;70(5):692–701.

37. Suggs JF, Li G, Park SE, et al. Function of the anterior cruciate ligament after unicompartmental knee arthroplasty: an in vitro robotic study. J Arthroplasty 2004;19(2):224–9.

38. Suggs JF, Li G, Park SE, et al. Knee biomechanics after UKA and its relation to the ACL–a robotic investigation. J Orthop Res 2006;24(4):588–94.

39. Hernigou P, Deschamps G. Posterior slope of the tibial implant and the outcome of unicompartmental knee arthroplasty. J Bone Joint Surg Am 2004;86-A(3):506–11.

40. Engh GA, Ammeen D. Is an intact anterior cruciate ligament needed in order to have a well-functioning unicondylar knee replacement? Clin Orthop Relat Res 2004;(428):170–3.

41. Lohmander LS, Englund PM, Dahl LL, et al. The long-term consequence of anterior cruciate ligament and meniscus injuries: osteoarthritis. Am J Sports Med 2007;35(10):1756–69.

42. Weston-Simons JS, Pandit H, Jenkins C, et al. Outcome of combined unicompartmental knee replacement and combined or sequential anterior cruciate ligament reconstruction: a study of 52 cases with mean follow-up of five years. J Bone Joint Surg Br 2012;94(9):1216–20.

43. Tinius M, Hepp P, Becker R. Combined unicompartmental knee arthroplasty and anterior cruciate ligament reconstruction. Knee Surg Sports Traumatol Arthrosc 2012;20(1):81–7.

44. Pandit H, Van Duren BH, Gallagher JA, et al. Combined anterior cruciate reconstruction and Oxford unicompartmental knee arthroplasty: in vivo kinematics. Knee 2008;15(2):101–6.

45. Citak M, Bosscher MR, Citak M, et al. Anterior cruciate ligament reconstruction after unicompartmental knee arthroplasty. Knee Surg Sports Traumatol Arthrosc 2011;19(10):1683–8.
46. Beard DJ, Pandit H, Gill HS, et al. The influence of the presence and severity of pre-existing patellofemoral degenerative changes on the outcome of the Oxford medial unicompartmental knee replacement. J Bone Joint Surg Br 2007;89(12): 1597–601.
47. Beard DJ, Pandit H, Ostlere S, et al. Pre-operative clinical and radiological assessment of the patellofemoral joint in unicompartmental knee replacement and its influence on outcome. J Bone Joint Surg Br 2007;89(12):1602–7.
48. Price AJ, Waite JC, Svard U. Long-term clinical results of the medial Oxford unicompartmental knee arthroplasty. Clin Orthop Relat Res 2005;(435):171–80.
49. Heyse TJ, Khefacha A, Cartier P. UKA in combination with PFR at average 12-year follow-up. Arch Orthop Trauma Surg 2010;130(10):1227–30.
50. Palumbo BT, Henderson ER, Edwards PK, et al. Initial experience of the Journey-Deuce bicompartmental knee prosthesis: a review of 36 cases. The Journal of arthroplasty 2011;26(6 Suppl):40–5.
51. Bruni D, Iacono F, Raspugli G, et al. Is unicompartmental arthroplasty an acceptable option for spontaneous osteonecrosis of the knee? Clin Orthop Relat Res 2012;470(5):1442–51.
52. Heyse TJ, Khefacha A, Fuchs-Winkelmann S, et al. UKA after spontaneous osteonecrosis of the knee: a retrospective analysis. Arch Orthop Trauma Surg 2011;131(5):613–7.
53. Parratte S, Argenson JN, Dumas J, et al. Unicompartmental knee arthroplasty for avascular osteonecrosis. Clin Orthop Relat Res 2007;464:37–42.

Arthroscopic Debridement of Unicompartmental Arthritis
Fact or Fiction?

Ahmad Badri, DO[a,b,c], Joseph Burkhardt, DO[d,e,*]

KEYWORDS

- Unicompartmental • Arthritis • Arthroscopy • Knee • Osteochondral
- Autologous chondrocyte implantation

KEY POINTS

- The choice of procedure should have a viable backup plan with a high-percentage outcome.
- Be conservative. A little bit of bad cartilage is better than none.
- Preserve options for future consideration.
- Treatment should be age matched. The benefits of a complex surgery in age groups likely to proceed on and requiring replacement need to be considered.
- Treatment of chondral abnormalities in all age groups younger than 40 years of age seems to have similar results. In those older than 40 years, these results are less predictable. Incorporating the realistic expectations of the patient in conjunction with time constraints and recovery needs to be discussed and considered before proceeding.

INTRODUCTION

Treating arthritis in the knee has been a challenge for doctors for many years. According to the US Centers for Disease Control and Prevention, arthritis is the leading cause of disability in the United States[1] and the cost to treat it is continuously increasing. Therefore, there is a constant effort to find new ways to treat the symptoms and delay the progression of this disease. Arthritis of the knee can range from involving 1 compartment of the knee to the 3 compartments of the knee, called tricompartmental arthritis. Unicompartmental arthritis of the knee is a degenerative condition that involves the medial or lateral aspect of the tibiofemoral joint. The most common

[a] Department of Orthopedics, Jersey City Medical Center, 355 Grand Street, Jersey City, NJ 07032, USA; [b] Department of Orthopedics, Meadowlands Hospital Medical Center, 55 Meadowlands Parkway, Secaucus, NJ, USA; [c] Touro COM, Harlem, NY, USA; [d] Michigan State University, East Lansing, MI, USA; [e] Department of Orthopedics, Bronsone Battle Creek Hospital, Bronson Battle, MI, USA
* Corresponding author.
E-mail address: jeburkh@aol.com

Clin Sports Med 33 (2014) 23–41
http://dx.doi.org/10.1016/j.csm.2013.08.008
0278-5919/14/$ – see front matter © 2014 Elsevier Inc. All rights reserved.

symptom of arthritis in the knee is pain, which may be caused by articular cartilage defects, meniscal disorders, ligamentous disorders, or a combination of these. Other symptoms may include stiffness, swelling, instability, and crepitus. The challenge in treating articular cartilage defects is that the cartilage cannot regenerate, and, after conservative management has failed, there are several surgical treatment options depending on the extent of disease and its involvement. Treatment options include debridement, lavage, chondroplasty, bone marrow–stimulating techniques, chondrocyte transfer, and chondrocyte implantation.

UNDERSTANDING ARTICULAR CARTILAGE

Articular cartilage is a highly specialized tissue that contains no blood supply or nerve tissue. Intact articular cartilage is commonly called hyaline cartilage and is composed of chondrocytes within an extracellular matrix of proteoglycans, collagen, and 80% water.[2–4] Most of the collagen is type 2, and the fibers are firmly imbedded in the subchondral bone.[3,5] As seen in **Fig. 1**, the superficial layer of cartilage has a high collagen content with low levels of proteoglycans and provides a smooth, gliding surface for the joint.[3,6] Deeper in the cartilage, the collagen content decreases along with decreasing amounts of water, whereas the proteoglycan content increases.[3,6] If the proteoglycans are damaged by trauma or other mechanisms such as inflammation, the structure disintegrates and the ability to hold water is reduced significantly. This condition leads to a breakdown of the collagen meshwork, which reduces the ability of cartilage to withstand compressive forces.[3,5] The deepest zone of cartilage is composed of calcified cartilage with a mineralized matrix.[3,6]

Cartilage initially receives nutrients through blood perfusion from subchondral bone during early childhood. As the calcified zone forms during skeletal maturation, flow of nutrients from subchondral bone is inhibited and cartilage becomes dependent on diffusion of nutrients from the joint cavity.[4]

This avascularity renders the cartilage unable to mount an inflammatory response to injury, unless the subchondral bone is also injured.[3,6] This result may also help to explain why repair tissue often degenerates over time. The repair tissue frequently

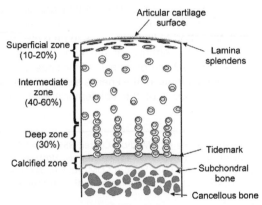

Fig. 1. Main zones of articular cartilage organization. Chondrocytes are elongated in the superficial zone, gradually become rounded, are repeatedly arranged in columns, and are surrounded by the extracellular matrix in deeper zones. (*From* Simon T, Jackson D. Articular cartilage: injury pathways and treatment options. Sports Med Arthrosc 2006;14:146–54; with permission.)

differs in its biomechanical properties and also may not be able to absorb nutrients through diffusion.[2,3] Although young individuals possess chondrocytes that maintain high metabolic rates and divide rapidly as skeletal maturity is reached, the cellular processes of chondrocytes slow and they divide less frequently, further reducing their capacity for healing.

There are several clinical problems in trying to duplicate or regenerate native articular cartilage. Articular cartilage forms embryologically from mesenchymal cells that cluster together and begin to synthesize a surrounding matrix.[3] These cells become more organized and are recognized as cartilage when they accumulate the matrix that separates the cells. The cells progressively take on their more characteristic spherical shape.[3,7] As the cartilage matures, there is a lack of multipotential cells and the new chondrocytes lose their ability to migrate, proliferate, and participate in a repair response. These characteristics limit the healing potential of articular cartilage.[3,7]

Treating an articular cartilage defect is multifactorial because the damage can vary in size, shape, depth, and location. Therefore treatment must take into account these variations as well as the patient's age, activity level, and associated conditions. Treatment options include, but are not limited to, arthroscopic debridement and lavage, bone-stimulation techniques, articular cartilage transplantation, osteochondral autograft transplantation (OAT), and osteochondral allograft transplantation.

CLASSIFYING ARTICULAR CARTILAGE

There are various classifications in the literature regarding the macroscopic changes of the patellofemoral and tibiofemoral joints. Of these, two widely used classifications are the Outerbridge classification (**Table 1**) and the International Cartilage Research Society (ICRS) grades (**Fig. 2, Table 2**).

The Outerbridge classification was initially used to describe the macroscopic changes of chondromalacia of the patella, but over time it has been adopted to describe the changes of the femoral condyles as well. There are 4 grades in this classification. In grade 1 there is softening and swelling of the cartilage. In grade 2 there is fragmentation and fissuring in an area 12 mm or less in diameter. Grade 3 is the same as grade 2, but the area involved is greater than 12 mm. In grade 4 there is eburnation or erosion of the cartilage down to bone.

The ICRS also describes 4 grades but with grade 0 being normal and grade 1 showing the initial changes of superficial lesions, fissures, and indentations. Grade 2 describes fraying of the cartilage and lesions less than 50% of the cartilage depth, and grade 3 describes lesions greater than 50% of the cartilage depth. Grade 4 is a complete loss of cartilage and exposure of the underlying bone.

Table 1	
Outerbridge classification	
Grade	**Description**
I	Softening and swelling
II	Fragmentation/fissuring <1.3 mm (0.5 in)
III	Fragmentation/fissuring >1.3 mm (0.5 in)
IV	Exposure of subchondral bone

Data from Outerbridge RE. The etiology of chondromalacia patellae. J Bone Joint Surg Br 1961;43: 752–7.

ICRS Grade 0 - Normal

ICRS Grade 1 – Nearly Normal

Superficial lesions. Soft indentation (A) and/or superficial fissures and cracks (B)

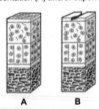

A   B

ICRS Grade 2 – Abnormal

Lesions extending down to <50% of cartilage depth

ICRS Grade 3 – Severely Abnormal

Cartilage defects extending down >50% of cartilage depth (A) as well as down to calcified layer (B) and down to but not through the subchondral bone (C). Blisters are included in this Grade (D)

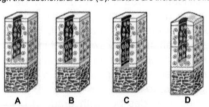

A   B   C   D

ICRS Grade 4 – Severely Abnormal

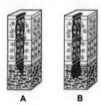

A   B

Fig. 2. ICRS articular cartilage grades. (*Courtesy of* International Cartilage Repair Society, Zurich, Switzerland; with permission. Available at: http://www.cartilage.org/_files/contentmanagement/ICRS_evaluation.pdf. Accessed February 13, 2013.)

HISTORY OF ARTHROSCOPY IN THE KNEE

The use of arthroscopy dates back to 1912 when a Danish surgeon, Severin Nordentoft, presented an article on endoscopic findings within the knee using a technique that

Table 2 ICRS	
Grade	Description
0	Normal
1	Superficial lesions, fissures, indentations
2	Fraying, lesions <50% of cartilage depth
3	Cartilage defects >50% of cartilage depth
4	Complete loss of cartilage thickness with exposed bone

Courtesy of International Cartilage Repair Society, Zurich, Switzerland; with permission. Available at: http://www.cartilage.org/_files/contentmanagement/ICRS_evaluation.pdf. Accessed February 13, 2013.

he named arthroscopy, as seen in **Fig. 3**. Several years later, several attempts at creating an ideal scope, capable of visualizing the joint and being minimally invasive, led to the development of the no. 1 arthroscope in 1931. This arthroscope, a 3.5-mm instrument, became the model for present-day instruments. In the same year, an American surgeon, Dr Michael Burmann, published the results of his investigation in the historic article, "Arthroscopy or the Direct Visualization of Joints," and created the first pictures of arthroscopic findings ever published. Then, in 1974, Dr Richard O'Conner performed the first partial meniscectomy in North America, and this was also the year the International Arthroscopy Association (IAA) was founded.[8] The IAA and the International Society of the Knee (ISK) merged in 1995 to become the International Society for Arthroscopy, Knee Surgery and Orthopaedic Sports Medicine (ISAKOS).

Arthroscopy of a painful arthritic knee permits a surgeon to define the extent of degenerative disease, formulate a treatment plan based on those findings, and correct mechanical problems that are responsive to arthroscopic treatment.[9,10]

DEBRIDEMENT AND LAVAGE

Arthroscopic debridement and lavage have been used since the 1940s as a means to treat symptoms caused by degenerative joint disease in the knee. The theory behind

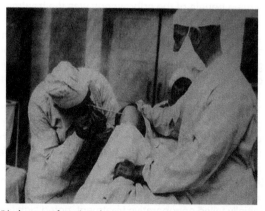

Fig. 3. Dr Eugen Bircher performing knee surgery with his arthroscope in 1917. (*From* Kieser CW, Jackson RW. Eugen Bircher (1882-1956) the first knee surgeon to use diagnostic arthroscopy. Arthroscopy 2003;19(7):771–6.)

doing a joint lavage was, in part, that the detachment of cartilage components that act as proinflammatory mediators causes synovitis. By diluting and removing these mediators there is potential for relief.[4] The goal of debridement of chondral defects is to remove any loose flaps of articular cartilage and to create a stable rim of intact cartilage, leading to reduced mechanical stresses.[11]

In a prospective review of 254 patients treated by arthroscopic knee debridement for osteoarthritis (OA) by Aichroth and colleagues,[12] 75% of patients had minimal discomfort after surgery and improved function. Further, almost 85% were satisfied with the treatment at an average follow-up of 44 months. These patients had more worthwhile improvement with less radiographic arthritis after undergoing arthroscopic debridement.

In a study to evaluate the effect of lavage, Edelson and colleagues[13] evaluated 29 knees of 23 patients with symptomatic arthritis and underwent washout with lactated Ringer solution. Results showed that 25 of these 29 knees had good to excellent results at 1 year, and 21 knees had good to excellent results at 2 years. The investigators concluded that there is some value in a fluid washout in an arthritic knee.

Although lavage may be involved in relieving pain in arthritic knees, it was only seen as a temporary relief by other studies. One such study was done on patients with moderate to severe arthritis by Kirkley and colleagues.[14] Patients were randomized into 2 groups: surgical lavage and arthroscopic debridement with physical and medical therapy versus nonoperative treatment, including physical and medical therapy only. Patients with large symptomatic meniscal tears were excluded from the study. The results showed that, at 3 months, the arthroscopic group had slightly better outcomes, but at 2 years no statistically significant clinical difference was noted between the groups.

Gibson and colleagues[15] conducted a study with similar results. They did a prospective study using 20 patients with moderate unilateral OA of the knee and allocated them randomly to treatment by either arthroscopic lavage or debridement and measured flexor and extensor muscle strength using biopsies. They concluded that there was some temporary relief in the lavage group as well as improvement in contractile properties of the muscle groups, but neither method significantly relieved patients' symptoms.

Merchant and Galindo[16] were among the first investigators to prospectively compare arthroscopic debridement with partial meniscectomy and chondroplasty of loose flaps to nonoperative treatment. In limited degenerative OA with normal limb alignment, the operative group did much better at short-term follow-up. They concluded that the main benefit of the arthroscopy was the treatment of concomitant problems that coexist with the OA, mainly symptomatic meniscus tears.

To further study the effect of meniscal tears in conjunction with OA, Herrlin and colleagues[17] conducted a prospective randomized trial for degenerative meniscus tears by allocating patients to arthroscopic partial meniscectomy in one group and treatment by exercise alone in the other group. Patients treated with arthroscopic partial meniscectomy and those treated with exercise alone had decreased pain, improved knee function, and a high rate of satisfaction with the treatment. The results between the two groups were similar for all outcomes at 6-month follow-up.

In a recently published 5-year follow-up on this patient cohort, Herrlin and colleagues[18] maintained comparable results with no significant differences between the patients treated with arthroscopy and those treated with exercise. However, one-third of the patients treated with exercise alone eventually received arthroscopic partial meniscectomy because of their pain. After arthroscopic partial meniscectomy, this group, which had initially failed nonoperative treatment, noted significant improvement.

The indications for this procedure are specific and there has been no evidence to suggest that it alters the pathologic process. For the properly selected patient, the rationale for offering arthroscopic debridement is that it may improve symptoms and function, has minimal morbidity, provides a temporizing therapeutic procedure, documents the stage of disease process, and is an attempt to delay the need for more invasive procedures such as joint replacement.[10,11,19]

Mechanical symptoms that may cause a popping or clicking on physical examination because of meniscal tears, loose bodies, osteophytic spurs, or chondral flaps can be treated successfully with this arthroscopic procedure.[10]

Therefore, in unicompartmental arthritis, arthroscopy can provide a clinical benefit in terms of reduced pain, improved functions in patients with mechanical symptoms, with minimal or no malalignment, for an indefinite period of time until further treatment can be done.[10,11,16,20,21]

BONE MARROW–STIMULATION TECHNIQUES

Marrow-stimulation techniques for treating chondral defects include chondroplasty, drilling, and microfracture. The underlying assumption behind marrow-stimulating techniques is that debriding the damaged cartilage and perforating the subchondral bone leads to a physiologic repair response. This repair response allows the blood and marrow elements to form a blood clot in the area of the defect. This blood clot, which contains mesenchymal cells, differentiates into fibrocartilage, which fills the defect. Fibrocartilage, type 1 collagen, exhibits inferior wear characteristics and does not resist compression and shear loads compared with hyaline cartilage, a type 2 collagen.[11]

Chondroplasty is achieved either mechanically by a shaver or burr (**Fig. 4**), or thermally by radiofrequency energy (RFE). It is done by removing the superficial layer and

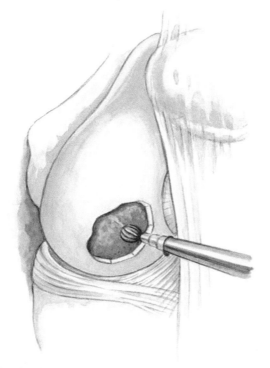

Fig. 4. Abrasion chondroplasty with a ball-shaped burr.

allowing for the exposure of the subchondral bone, depending on the depth of the defect.[4]

Microfracture is a procedure introduced by Steadman more than 20 years ago as a modification of the Pridie[22] drilling technique. It includes debridement of all unstable and damaged articular cartilage, down to the subchondral bone plate, while maintaining a stable perpendicular edge of healthy cartilage. An arthroscopic awl is used to make multiple holes, about 3 to 4 mm apart in the defect, ensuring that the subchondral plate is kept intact (**Figs. 5** and **6**). At this point, if a tourniquet is being used it should be released to allow blood flow into the microfracture sites. The defect fills with hematoma (**Fig. 7**), producing an environment for pluripotential marrow cells to differentiate into fibrocartilage.[20] Advantages of microfracture compared with drilling may include reduced thermal damage to subchondral bone and the creation of a rougher surface to which repair tissue might adhere more easily.[20]

The best results of microfracture are seen with successful completion of the vigorous rehabilitation program. It consists of cold therapy, continuous passive motion (CPM) use, and strength training, a few days to weeks following surgery. Once patients obtain full range of motion and adequate pain control they begin assisted crutch training for 6 to 8 weeks, which may be in combination with deep water exercises. Patients then progress to full weight bearing after 8 weeks and begin the more rigorous use of the knee, including an elastic resistance cord and then free/machine weights 16 weeks later. According to Steadman and Briggs,[23] "the rehabilitation program promotes the optimal physical environment for the mesenchymal stem cells to differentiate

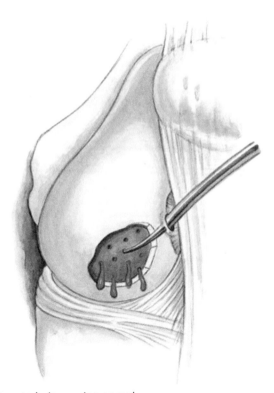

Fig. 5. Microfracture technique using an awl.

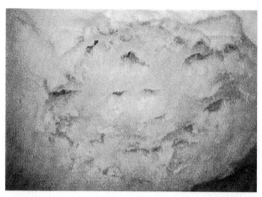

Fig. 6. After thorough debridement an awl is used to make multiple holes, about 3 to 4 mm apart.

and produce new extracellular matrix that eventually matures into a durable repair tissue. This is the basis for the next most ideal chemical environment to complement the physical environment."

Steadman and colleagues[24] conducted a study on 75 knees that underwent microfracture and followed them for an average of 11 years to measure functional outcomes. Patients ranged between the ages of 13 and 45 years and had no associated meniscal or ligament injuries. At 7 to 17 years after surgery, 80% of the patients rated themselves as improved. The investigators concluded that over the 7-year to 17-year follow-up period, patients up to 45 years of age who underwent microfracture for isolated chondral defects showed statistically significant improvement in function and pain.

Arthroscopic microfracture of subchondral bone can be safe and effective for initial treatment of full-thickness chondral defects of the knee. It has been shown to improve functional outcomes and decrease pain in most patients. Therefore full-thickness chondral lesions, acute or chronic, less than 4 cm^2 respond better to microfracture than those lesions greater than 4 cm^2.[24,25]

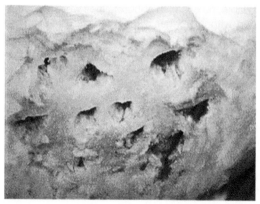

Fig. 7. With release of the tourniquet, blood flow should be seen and allowed to form a clot.

Mechanical/Thermal Chondroplasty

Damaged cartilage causes the release of inflammatory cytokines and the formation of synovitis, creating rough surfaces that lead to crepitus and pain. The aim of chondroplasty therefore is to create a smooth edge without damaging the surrounding cartilage, and this can be done either with a mechanical shaver or by using RFE.

Mechanical chondroplasty causes a cutting or tearing effect on the cartilage surface, making it difficult to achieve a smooth surface. The rough edge is susceptible to further degradation by cyclical forces and recurrence of the fibrillation.[26]

The use of RFE to perform arthroscopic chondroplasty in the knee has become increasingly popular. RFE stabilizes the chondral lesion, seals fibrillation, and gives a macroscopically smoother edge.[26]

Initial concerns with the use of RFE for chondroplasty were from research suggesting that it may cause osteonecrosis, damage to surrounding cartilage, and progression of partial-thickness lesions. However, in a study by Cetik and colleagues[27] on 50 patients undergoing bipolar RFE chondroplasty for Outerbridge 2 and 3 lesions, findings showed that only 2 patients had magnetic resonance imaging (MRI) findings of osteonecrosis. The investigators concluded that bipolar RFE used for arthroscopic chondroplasty does not cause osteonecrosis if proper surgical techniques are performed.

In a study of 60 patients,[28] 30 were treated with mechanical shaving and the other 30 were treated with mechanical shaving plus monopolar frequency. On the posttreatment MRI study obtained 12 months after surgery, there was no evidence of heat-related subchondral damage such as avascular necrosis. The mean 19-month clinical data did not show any effect from the addition of monopolar radiofrequency (MRF) to the treatment of grade III chondral lesions. Both treatment with the mechanical shaver alone and treatment with the mechanical shaver plus MRF resulted in significant improvements in pain.

Lu and colleagues[29] published a study regarding the effects of RFE on articular cartilage. This study used a monopolar device on sheep articular cartilage and showed full-thickness articular cartilage necrosis at time zero and at 6 months. The same investigators then conducted a second study using a live cell-dead cell assay at time zero to determine the viability of human articular cartilage treated with bipolar RFE. Bipolar RFE resulted in full-thickness red staining and the investigators concluded that this indicated that the entire thickness of cartilage and adjacent bone was dead.[30] These findings are questionable because live/dead cell assays can overstimulate cell death by 50%.[31,32] A similar study was done by Kaplan and Uribe[33] in which chondrocytes were treated with RFE using tissue dye and histologic techniques. The chondrocytes remained viable, no collagen abnormalities were detected, and the diseased areas were smoothed without further evidence of fibrillation. They showed that the morphologic and histologic appearance of the cartilage is superior after radiofrequency debridement.[33] Evidence suggests increased mechanical stability, decreased release of inflammatory mediators, decreased postoperative pain, and superior clinical outcomes compared with mechanical shaving.[34–37]

The use of thermal chondroplasty to treat articular cartilage defects in the knee is controversial. In other applications in the knee, it has been used in anterior cruciate ligament (ACL)/posterior cruciate ligament site preparation, for ACL guidewire placement, and in patellofemoral instability.

ADVANCED CARTILAGE REPAIR TECHNIQUES
Autologous Chondrocyte Implantation

Autologous chondrocyte implantation (ACI) is a 2-step procedure (**Fig. 8**) that introduces chondrogenic cells containing hyaline cartilage into the chondral defect. The

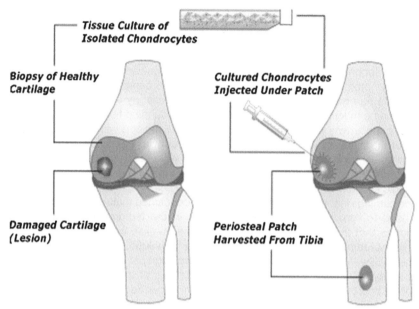

Tissue Culture of Isolated Chondrocytes

Biopsy of Healthy Cartilage

Cultured Chondrocytes Injected Under Patch

Damaged Cartilage (Lesion)

Periosteal Patch Harvested From Tibia

Fig. 8. The 2-step procedure of ACI, which may or may not include a periosteal patch harvested from the tibia.

first step is an arthroscopic procedure that consists of evaluation of the lesion and harvesting a cartilage biopsy of 200 to 300 mg, which contains around 200,000 to 300,000 chondrocytes. These cells are allowed to expand in a monolayer culture for several weeks to create millions of cells, depending on the size of the initial defect.

The second step usually occurs about 2 to 6 weeks after biopsy, when the cells are reimplanted into the chondral defect through an arthrotomy. The defect is prepared by debridement down to the calcific zone of any fibrocartilage that may have formed. Next, a periosteal patch is harvested from the proximal medial part of the tibia, and is sewn to the cartilage. However, in more recent studies, the periosteal patch has been a cause of complication and is left out, and instead the implanted cartilage is sutured down.

In a study to evaluate the overall long-term results of ACI, Moradi and colleagues[38] used several parameters to evaluate this procedure, including patient satisfaction and MRI. The study evaluated 23 patients with full-thickness chondral lesions for up to 14 years, during which patients underwent MRI before surgery and at various intervals. The investigators reported substantial improvement in all clinical outcome parameters. MRI findings confirmed complete defect filling in about 52% of the patients at final follow-up.

Brittberg and colleagues[39,40] performed ACI on 23 patients with a mean age of 27 years and a mean follow-up time of 39 months. Ten of these patients had previously undergone arthroscopic debridement of fibrillated cartilage and unstable chondral flaps with a brief improvement in symptoms. Seven of these 27 patients had defects of the patellar facet caused by either chondromalacia (grade IV lesion) or, in 1 case, a defect of traumatic origin.

After the initial surgery was performed, the collected cells were grown in a culture for 14 to 21 days before transplantation. Evaluation included a clinical examination based on their criteria as well as postoperative arthroscopic examination with a biopsy of the transplantation site.

At 3 months, arthroscopy showed that transplants were level with the surrounding tissue and spongy when probed, with visible borders. At about 12 months, 2 patients required a second surgery because of locking of the knee and pain, but 6 months after surgery symptoms improved. At 2 years, 14 of the 16 patients with femoral condylar transplants had good to excellent results and arthroscopy showed that transplants had the same macroscopic appearance as the surrounding tissue.

Biopsy specimens were obtained from 15 of the 16 patients with femoral transplants and 7 of the patellar transplants. In the femoral condylar transplant, 11 patients had intact articular surface and a hyaline appearance, whereas only 1 of the patellar transplants had the same appearance; the remaining 6 had areas of irregular fibrous tissue. Histologic sections indicated that the transplanted cells were regenerated into normal hyaline cartilage in the defect. The investigators concluded that ACI could be successfully used to repair articular cartilage defects in the femorotibial joint. They also concluded that the treatment of chondromalacia patellae was less successful than treatment of femoral condylar defects using this technique.[39]

When ACI was compared with debridement, although patients treated with debridement for symptomatic, large, focal, chondral defects of the distal femur had some functional improvement at follow-up, patients who received ACI obtained higher levels of knee function and had greater relief from pain and swelling at 3 years.[41]

Patients with moderate to large chondral lesions with failed prior cartilage treatments can expect sustained and clinically meaningful improvement in pain and function after ACI. This finding was shown by Zaslav and colleagues,[42] who took 154 patients with failed treatments of articular cartilage defects of the knee and had ACI done to determine whether ACI provided a clinical benefit in patients with failed prior articular cartilage treatments. Patients were followed up for 48 months and outcomes were determined based on change from baseline knee function, knee pain, quality of life, and overall health. Of the 126 patients who completed the study, 76% were deemed treatment successes and 24% were deemed treatment failures. These results did not differ between patients whose primary surgery was a marrow-stimulating procedure and those who had only debridement.

The tissue that was generated in ACI was superior to the tissue generated in microfracture.[43] This tissue was tested in a study evaluating 61 patients after ACI for a mean follow-up of 7.4 years, and in some patients for up to 11 years. They took biopsies of the graft site for 12 of these patients through a second arthroscopy and tested the graft site for hyaline using safranin O staining. Eight of the 12 patients tested positive for hyalinelike species and the remaining 3 tested positive for fibrocartilage. The investigators concluded that ACI for the treatment of articular cartilage injuries may produce hyaline cartilage in the defect and has a durable outcome for as long as 11 years,[44] and in other studies[45] for up to 20 years.

Although the results of ACI are viable and promising, it is a 2-stage procedure that is laboratory dependent, requires an arthrotomy, and may be more expensive than other techniques mentioned earlier. It can also be associated with resultant pain and catching caused by the hypertrophic periosteal healing.[46]

Osteochondral Grafting

Osteochondral autograft transplantation (OAT) is used in procedures such as the osteochondral autograft transfer system (OATS) and mosaicplasty to address medium-sized defects (1–4 cm). In this technique, cartilage and subchondral bone are harvested from lesser or non–weight-bearing areas of the knee, such as the periphery of the femoral condyles or intercondylar notch, and transferred to the weight-bearing area containing the chondral defect. Depending on the size of the defect, either a single or multiple cylinders may have to be transplanted to fill a larger defect. This procedure allows for the transplantation of viable hyaline cartilage in a single operation (**Figs. 9** and **10**).

In a retrospective study to evaluate the results of arthroscopic treatment of articular cartilage lesions, Chow and Hantes[47] evaluated 33 patients with full-thickness lesions, 1 to 2.5 cm^2, of the femoral condyle using osteochondral autograft for an average period of 45 months. All patients were evaluated with the Lysholm knee and International Knee Documentation Committee (IKDC) standard evaluation form before and after surgery and results show an increase in the mean scores of both Lysholm and IKDC. Repeat arthroscopy with needle biopsy was performed on 9 patients and histology revealed viable chondrocytes and normal hyaline cartilage. Marcacci and colleagues[48] similarly did a prospective study to evaluate mosaicplasty on active patients with grade III to IV lesions (less than 2.5 cm) of the lateral condyle via arthroscopy. At an average of 2 years' follow-up they had 78% clinically satisfactory results. When an MRI was done at about 7 years, they found good integration of the graft in the host bone and complete maintenance of the grafted cartilage in more than 60% of the cases.[49] In another study investigating articular cartilage lesions in physically active athletes, Gudas and colleagues[50] evaluated 60 athletes less than 40 years of age with a symptomatic lesion of the articular cartilage in the knee who were randomized to undergo either OATS or microfracture (MF) and were followed for about 38 months. According to the modified hospital of special surgery (HSS) and ICRS scores, functional and objective assessment showed that 96% had excellent or good results after OAT compared with 52% for the MF procedure. They concluded that in this population there was a significant superiority of OAT compared with MF for the repair of articular cartilage defects in the knee.

OAT mosaicplasty, done either in a minimally invasive incision or arthroscopically, can alleviate knee pain and improve knee functionality in properly selected patients. Studies have shown that it is an effective technique for restoration of articular cartilage lesions of the femoral condyles, especially in active patients.[48,50]

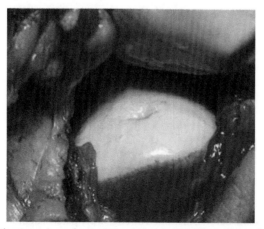

Fig. 9. After an arthrotomy is performed the defect is identified. (*From* Gomoll A, Yanke A, Cole B. Articular cartilage lesion. In: DeLee JC, David Drez D, Miller MD, eds. Delee and Drez's orthopaedic sports medicine. Philadelphia: Elsevier Saunders, 2010; with permission.)

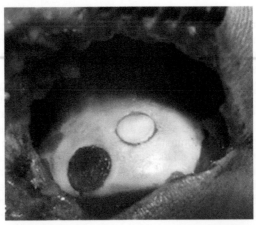

Fig. 10. An osteochondral autograft is removed from the lesser weight-bearing area, transferred to the identified defect, and the harvest site is covered with a synthetic plug. (*From* Gomoll A, Yanke A, Cole B. Articular cartilage lesion. In: DeLee JC, David Drez D, Miller MD, eds. Delee and Drez's orthopaedic sports medicine. Philadelphia: Elsevier Saunders, 2010; with permission.)

Osteochondral allograft transplantation is used predominantly in the treatment of larger defects (3–7 cm) and as a salvage option after failure of other cartilage resurfacing procedures. By using an allograft, there is a closer match of the geometric curvature of the articular cartilage from the cadaver to the donor, compared with other procedures. This technique can be done arthroscopically or via arthrotomy depending on the size and location of the defect (**Figs. 11–14**).

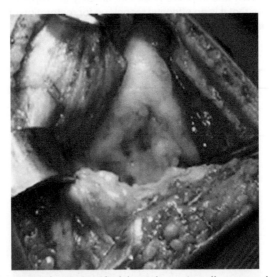

Fig. 11. A large chondral defect is identified through a peripatellar approach. (*From* Gomoll A, Yanke A, Cole B. Articular cartilage lesion. In: DeLee JC, David Drez D, Miller MD, eds. Delee and Drez's orthopaedic sports medicine. Philadelphia: Elsevier Saunders, 2010; with permission.)

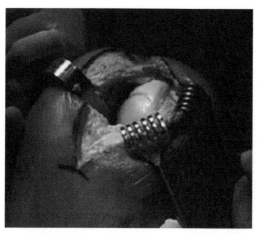

Fig. 12. The defect is prepared by debridement and reaming to about 6 to 8 mm. (*From* Gomoll A, Yanke A, Cole B. Articular cartilage lesion. In: DeLee JC, David Drez D, Miller MD, eds. Delee and Drez's orthopaedic sports medicine. Philadelphia: Elsevier Saunders, 2010; with permission.)

OUTCOMES OF OSTEOCHONDRAL ALLOGRAFT TRANSPLANTATION

Chahal and colleagues[51] conducted a systematic review of clinical outcomes after osteochondral allograft transplantation in the knee and reviewed more than 400 studies using certain inclusion criteria and narrowed it down to 19 studies they considered eligible. Of these 19 eligible studies there were 644 knees with a mean follow-up of 58 months. The mean age was 37 years and the mean defect size was 6.3 cm². Studies included a variety of allografts including fresh, prolonged fresh, and fresh frozen. Causes and defect locations included medial femoral condyle (n = 261), lateral femoral condyle (n = 142), patella (n = 45), tibial plateau (n = 77), and bipolar locations (n = 16). Several articles compared preoperative and postoperative scores and

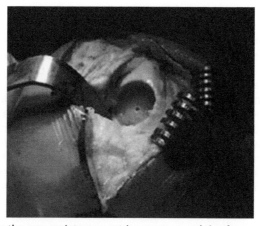

Fig. 13. Identifying the appropriate geometric curvature and size from a cadaveric condyle. (*From* Gomoll A, Yanke A, Cole B. Articular cartilage lesion. In: DeLee JC, David Drez D, Miller MD, eds. Delee and Drez's orthopaedic sports medicine. Philadelphia: Elsevier Saunders, 2010; with permission.)

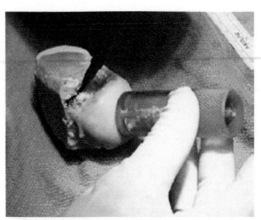

Fig. 14. The transplant is placed in the defect site and can either press fit or augmented with resorbable pins. (*From* Gomoll A, Yanke A, Cole B. Articular cartilage lesion. In: DeLee JC, David Drez D, Miller MD, eds. Delee and Drez's orthopaedic sports medicine. Philadelphia: Elsevier Saunders, 2010; with permission.)

several different functional outcome scores were used, including Lysholm, Tegner, IKDC, and Knee Injury and Osteoarthritis Outcome Score.

Fresh-frozen allografts showed significant postoperative Lysholm and Tegner (74 and 4, respectively) differences compared with the preoperative values (38 and 2, respectively).[52]

In the fresh allografts, Convery and colleagues[53] reported that unipolar lesions on the medial femoral condyle had excellent or good results in 86% and unipolar results of the lateral femoral condyle had excellent or good results in 88% of cases. Good results were also seen in the prolonged fresh allografts and results can be seen in the original article.[51]

The investigators concluded that, at a mean follow-up of 5 years, using allograft transplantation for focal and diffuse (single-compartment) chondral defects results in predictable favorable outcomes, high satisfaction rates (86%), and a low short-term complication rate (2.4%).

OVERVIEW

The goals of treatment are to alleviate pain, improve functionality, and delay the possibility of joint replacement, especially in younger active patients. Therefore each procedure should be age matched and should have a viable backup plan in case the results do not meet expectations.

Traditional resurfacing techniques, such as drilling and microfracture, have proved to be safe and effective for treating grade III to IV articular cartilage lesions of the knee of less than 2 to 3 cm^2 but do not restore normal hyaline cartilage and have short-term success rates. Newer techniques have been developed that provide hyaline or hyalinelike cartilage for the treatment of grade III to IV lesions that can treat larger defects and have longer success rates. These techniques, namely ACI and osteochondral grafting, provide viable and promising options, but they have limitations.

REFERENCES

1. Centers for Disease Control and Prevention CDC. Prevalence of disabilities and associated health conditions among adults—United States, 1999. MMWR Morb Mortal Wkly Rep 2001;50:120–5.

2. Newman AP. Articular cartilage repair. Am J Sports Med 1998;26:309–24.
3. Cooper MT, Miller M. Primary articular cartilage procedures in the middle-aged knee. Sports Med Arthrosc 2003;11:112–21.
4. Erggelet C, Mandelbaum B. Principles of cartilage repair. Germany: Steinkopff Verlag-Springer; 2008. p. 39–66.
5. Minas T, Nehrer S. Current concepts in the treatment of articular cartilage defects. Orthopedics 1997;20:525–38.
6. Buckwalter JA, Mankin HJ. Articular cartilage: tissue design and chondrocyte-matrix interactions. Instr Course Lect 1998;47:477–86.
7. Simon T, Jackson D. Articular cartilage: injury pathways and treatment options. Sports Med Arthrosc 2006;14:146–54.
8. Hans H, Yuping Y. The past and the future of Arthroscopy. Springer; 2012.
9. Stuart MJ. Arthroscopic management for degenerative arthritis of the knee. Instr Course Lect 1999;48:135–41.
10. Iorio R, Healey W. Current concepts review: unicompartmental arthritis of the knee. J Bone Joint Surg Am 2003;85(7):1351–64.
11. Gomoll A, Yanke A, Cole B. Delee and Dresz's orthopaedic sports medicine: Ch 23; section I. p. 1771–86.
12. Aichroth PM, Patel DV, Moyes ST. A prospective review of arthroscopic débridement for degenerative joint disease of the knee. Int Orthop 1991;15:351–5.
13. Edelson R, Burks RT, Bloebaum RD. Short-term effects of knee washout for osteoarthritis. Am J Sports Med 1995;23:345–9.
14. Kirkley A, Birmingham TB, Litchfield RB, et al. A randomized trial of arthroscopic surgery for osteoarthritis of the knee. N Engl J Med 2008;359(11):1097–107.
15. Gibson JN, White MD, Chapman VM, et al. Arthroscopic lavage and débridement for osteoarthritis of the knee. J Bone Joint Surg Br 1992;74:534–7.
16. Merchan EC, Galindo E. Arthroscope-guided surgery versus nonoperative treatment for limited degenerative osteoarthritis of the femorotibial joint in patients over 50 years of age: a prospective comparative study. Arthroscopy 1993;9:663–7.
17. Herrlin S, Hallander M, Wange P, et al. Arthroscopic or conservative treatment of degenerative medial meniscal tears: a prospective randomized trial. Knee Surg Sports Traumatol Arthrosc 2007;15(4):393–401.
18. Herrlin S, Hallander M, Wange P, et al. Is arthroscopic surgery beneficial in treating non-traumatic, degenerative medial meniscal tears? A five year follow-up. Knee Surg Sports Traumatol Arthrosc 2013;21(2):358–64.
19. Timoney JM, Kneisl JS, Barrack RL, et al. Arthroscopy update #6. Arthroscopy in the osteoarthritic knee. Long term follow up. Orthop Rev 1990;19(4):371–3, 376–9.
20. Krishnan SP, Skinner J. Novel treatments for early osteoarthritis of the knee. Elsevier. Curr Orthop 2005;19:407–14.
21. Harwin S. Arthroscopic debridement for osteoarthritis of the knee: predictors of patient satisfaction. Arthroscopy 1999;15(2):142–6.
22. Pridie KH. A method of resurfacing osteoarthritic knee joints. J Bone Joint Surg Br 1959;41:618–9.
23. Steadman JR, Briggs KK. Outcomes of microfracture for traumatic chondral defects of the knee: average 11-year follow-up. Arthroscopy 2003;19:477–84.
24. Steadman JR, Rodkey W, Briggs K. Microfracture chondroplasty: indications, techniques, and outcomes. Sports Med Arthrosc 2003;11(4):236–44.
25. Knutsen G, Engebretsen L. Autologous chondrocyte implantation compared with microfracture in the knee. A randomized trial. J Bone Joint Surg Am 2004;86(3):455–64.

26. Kosy JD, Schranz PJ, Toms AD, et al. The use of radiofrequency energy for arthroscopic chondroplasty in the knee. Arthroscopy 2011;27(5):695–703.
27. Cetik O, Cift H, Comert B, et al. Risk of osteonecrosis of the femoral condyle after arthroscopic chondroplasty using radiofrequency: a prospective clinical series. Knee Surg Sports Traumatol Arthrosc 2009;17(1):24–9.
28. Barber FA, Iwasko N. Treatment of grade 3 femoral chondral lesions: mechanical chondroplasty versus monopolar radiofrequency probe. Arthroscopy 2006; 12:1312–7.
29. Lu Y, Hayashi K, Hecht P, et al. The effect of monopolar radiofrequency energy on partial-thickness defects of articular cartilage. Arthroscopy 2000;16: 527–36.
30. Lu Y, Edwards RB 3rd, Markel MD. Effect of bipolar radiofrequency energy on human articular cartilage. Comparison of confocal laser microscopy and light microscopy. Arthroscopy 2001;17:117–23.
31. Yetkinler DN, McCarthy EF. The use of live/dead cell viability stains with confocal microscopy in cartilage research. Sci Bull 2000;1:1–2.
32. Barber F, Uribe JW, Weber S. Current applications for arthroscopic thermal surgery. Arthroscopy 2002;18(2):40–50.
33. Kaplan L, Uribe JW. The acute effects of radiofrequency energy in articular cartilage: an in vitro study. Arthroscopy 2000;16(1):2–5.
34. Owens BD, Stickles BJ, Balikian P, et al. Prospective analysis of RF versus mechanical debridement of isolated patellar chondral lesions. Arthroscopy 2002; 18(2):151–5.
35. Voloshin I, Morse KR, Allred CD, et al. Arthroscopic evaluation of radiofrequency chondroplasty of the knee. Am J Sports Med 2007;35(10):1702–7.
36. Spahn G, Kahl E, Mückley T, et al. Arthroscopic knee chondroplasty using a bipolar RF based device compared to mechanical shaver: results of a prospective, randomized controlled study. Knee Surg Sports Traumatol Arthrosc 2008; 16(6):565–73.
37. Spahn G, Klinger HM, Mückley T, et al. Four-year results from a randomized controlled study of knee chondroplasty with concomitant medial meniscectomy: mechanical debridement versus RF chondroplasty. Arthroscopy 2008;16(6): 565–73.
38. Moradi B, Schonit E, Nierhoff C, et al. First-generation autologous chondrocyte implantation in patients with cartilage defects of the knee: 7-14 years clinical and MRI follow-up evaluation. Arthroscopy 2012;28:1851–61.
39. Brittberg M, Lindahl A, Nilsson A, et al. Treatment of deep cartilage defects in the knee with autologous chondrocyte transplantation. N Engl J Med 1994; 331:889–95.
40. Knutsen G, Drogset JO, Engebretsen L, et al. A randomized trial comparing autologous chondrocyte implantation with microfracture. Findings at five years. J Bone Joint Surg Am 2007;89:2105–12.
41. Fu F, Zurakowski D, Browne JE, et al. Autologous chondrocyte implantation versus debridement for treatment of full-thickness chondral defects of the knee: an observational cohort study with 3-year follow-up. Am J Sports Med 2005;33:1658–66.
42. Zaslav K, Cole B, Brewster R, et al, STAR Study Principal Investigators. A prospective study of autologous chondrocyte implantation in patients with failed prior treatment for articular cartilage defect of the knee: results of the Study of the Treatment of Articular Repair (STAR) clinical trial. Am J Sports Med 2009;37:42–55.

43. Saris DB, Vanlauwe J, Victor J. Characterized chondrocyte implantation results in better structural repair when treating symptomatic cartilage defects of the knee in a randomized controlled trial versus microfracture. Am J Sports Med 2008;36:235–46.
44. Peterson L, Brittberg M, Kiviranta I, et al. Autologous chondrocyte transplantation. Biomechanics and long-term durability. Am J Sports Med 2002;30:2–12.
45. Mahomed M, Beaver R, Gross A. The long-term success of fresh, small fragment osteochondral allografts used for intra-articular post-traumatic defects in the knee joint. Orthopedics 1992;15:1191–992.
46. Minas T, Peterson L. Advanced techniques in autologous chondrocyte transplantation. Clin Sports Med 1999;18:13–44.
47. Chow J, Hantes M. Arthroscopic autogenous osteochondral transplantation for treating knee cartilage defects: a 2- to 5-year follow-up study. Arthroscopy 2004; 20(7):681–90.
48. Marcacci M, Kon E, Zaffagnini S, et al. Multiple osteochondral arthroscopic grafting (mosaicplasty) for cartilage defects of the knee: prospective study results at 2-year follow-up. Arthroscopy 2005;21(4):462–70.
49. Marcacci M, Kon E, Delcogliano M, et al. Arthroscopic autologous osteochondral grafting for cartilage defects of the knee: prospective study results at a minimum 7-year follow-up. Am J Sports Med 2007;35:2014–21.
50. Gudas R, Kalesinskas RJ, Kimtys V, et al. A prospective randomized clinical study of mosaic osteochondral autologous transplantation versus microfracture for the treatment of osteochondral defects in the knee joint in young athletes. Arthroscopy 2005;21:1066–75.
51. Chahal J, Gross A, Gross C. Outcomes of osteochondral allograft transplantation in the knee. Arthroscopy 2013;29(3):575–88.
52. Karataglis D, Learmonth DJ. Management of big osteochondral defects of the knee using osteochondral allografts with the MEGA-OATS technique. Knee 2005;12:389–93.
53. Convery FR, Botte MJ, Akeson WH, et al. Chondral defects of the knee. Contemp Orthop 1994;28:101–7.

The Anterior Cruciate Ligament–Deficient Knee and Unicompartmental Arthritis

Kevin D. Plancher, MD, MS, FACS, FAAOS[a,b,c],*, Albert S.M. Dunn, DO[b],
Stephanie C. Petterson, PhD[b]

KEYWORDS

- Anterior cruciate ligament • ACL deficient • Unicompartmental arthritis
- Unicondylar arthroplasty • UKA • Coper • High tibial osteotomy • Pes bursitis

KEY POINTS

- Anterior cruciate ligament (ACL) insufficiency is not a contraindication for unicondylar knee arthroplasty (UKA).
- Fixed-bearing UKA may be successfully performed with long-term follow-up greater than 8 years in appropriately selected patients with ACL-deficient knees without the need for ACL reconstruction.
- Mobile-bearing UKA should be cautiously performed in patients with an ACL-deficient knee unless a previous or concomitant ACL reconstruction is performed.
- Maximize tibial component fixation; use the largest tibial tray possible without any overhang.
- A posterior tibial slope of less than 5° in ACL-deficient knees is associated with improved outcomes after UKA.
- Patients with a UKA without concomitant ACL reconstruction should expect intermittent pes bursitis for 6 months postoperatively; complete resolution of symptoms is expected.
- Fixed-bearing lateral UKA in the ACL-deficient knee is also successful but should not be attempted in the mobile-bearing knee.

INTRODUCTION

Management of medial and lateral compartment knee osteoarthritis (OA) in an anterior cruciate ligament (ACL)-deficient knee has remained a topic of controversy among orthopedic surgeons. Patient expectations and the desire to maintain a high level of pain-free activity complicate the decision making for this select group of patients.

[a] Plancher Orthopaedics & Sports Medicine, 1160 Park Avenue, New York, NY 10128, USA;
[b] Orthopaedic Foundation for Active Lifestyles, Greenwich, CT, USA; [c] Department of Orthopaedics, Albert Einstein College of Medicine, New York, NY, USA
* Corresponding author.
E-mail address: kplancher@plancherortho.com

Clin Sports Med 33 (2014) 43–55
http://dx.doi.org/10.1016/j.csm.2013.08.006
0278-5919/14/$ – see front matter © 2014 Elsevier Inc. All rights reserved.
sportsmed.theclinics.com

Treatment options have ranged from high tibial osteotomy (HTO) with and without ACL reconstruction to total knee arthroplasty (TKA).[1] Recent advances in surgical technique and prosthesis design have made unicondylar knee arthroplasty (UKA) a viable treatment option for the ACL-deficient, arthritic knee (**Fig. 1**).

TREATMENT OPTIONS
High Tibial Osteotomy

It has been well established that varus deformity of the knee can lead to progressive ligamentous laxity. The anatomic abnormalities of alignment, motion, joint position, and ligament defects associated with OA have been classified by Noyes as a single, double, or triple varus knee.[2]

The goal of HTO in the varus knee is to shift the mechanical axis of the knee laterally to decrease the load on the diseased, medial compartment. HTO can be performed with concomitant ACL reconstruction or with multiplane correction of varus angulation and tibial slope to decrease anterior tibial translation in the ACL-deficient knee with isolated medial compartment arthritis.[2] An intercondylar notchplasty is recommended

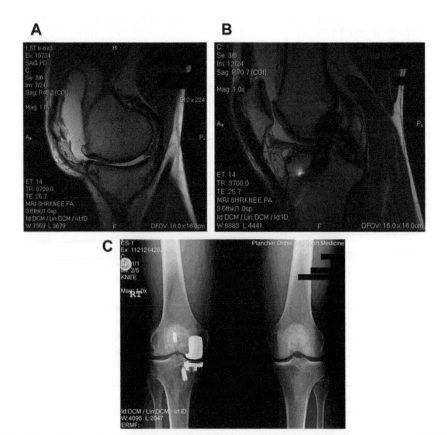

Fig. 1. (A) Magnetic resonance (MR) arthrogram sagittal proton density image of medial compartment OA in an ACL-deficient knee. (B) MR arthrogram sagittal proton density image of the same patient with a failed previous ACL reconstruction in a medial compartment osteoarthritic knee. (C) Postoperative plain radiograph of UKA in ACL-deficient knee in the same patient.

to avoid compromise of the graft and subsequent failure when performing a simultaneous ACL reconstruction and HTO.[3]

One of the drawbacks to HTO is the prolonged, protected weight bearing in the immediate postoperative period. Protection during this healing period negatively affects muscle strength and activation for as long as 1 year postoperatively[4] and potentially magnifies the functional deficits already present as a result of OA.

Although excellent results have been reported by experienced, high-volume surgeons, conflicting evidence is apparent in the literature. Despite survival rates of 98% after 5 years, 92% after 10 years, and 71% after 15 years,[5] high complication rates have also been reported (range 16%–21%).[6,7] In a recent study, 22% of patients undergoing combined ACL reconstruction and closing-wedge osteotomy showed significant progression of OA in the medial compartment 6.5 years postoperatively.[8] Another study reported that 25% of patients had not returned to their previous level of activity 25 months after simultaneous ACL reconstruction and HTO for ACL insufficiency and varus alignment.[9] Therefore, HTO may be a less desirable option for the middle-aged, active individual with an arthritic knee who wants to return to a high level of activity, particularly jumping and pivoting sports, because of poor patient satisfaction and continued pain with activities.[5,10]

Total Knee Arthroplasty

TKA is one of the most successful elective, orthopedic surgeries, resulting in pain relief and excellent survivorship for persons with either unicompartmental or tricompartmental disease.[11,12] Although other procedures for the ACL-deficient, arthritic knee may require some form of ACL reconstruction or osseous realignment, TKA relies entirely on the component design and positioning to provide stability. Although there is the rare component design that may substitute for the ACL, almost all other TKA designs are ACL deficient, either with deficiency present at time of surgery or via sacrifice of the ACL during the surgical procedure. As a result, kinematics of the knee after TKA are not similar to that of the native knee. Evidence suggests that abnormal movement patterns persist after TKA, which may compromise the health of other joints.[13–19]

TKA reliably reduces pain and increases activity level; however, patients report dissatisfaction with their activity level 1 year after surgery.[20] Polyethylene wear is also a concern after TKA. Premature wear has been associated with higher levels of postoperative activity, and therefore, it is recommended that patients avoid activities such as tennis and skiing to avoid stressing the knee and to minimize possible failure.[21] Consequently, patients, regardless of age, desiring an active lifestyle after surgery may be disappointed by the limitations set on them after TKA.[22]

Unicompartmental Knee Arthroplasty

Historically, UKA has not been a viable option for the ACL-deficient, arthritic knee and is still controversial. Concerns of poor survivorship and unpredictable outcomes limit its use in the ACL-deficient knee.

Kozinn and Scott[23] set forth selection criteria for successful UKA in their hallmark study in 1989. They indicated that ACL deficiency in addition to inflammatory arthritis, age younger than 60 years, high activity level, and patellofemoral pain or pain not isolated to the affected compartment are contraindications for UKA. Indications of successful UKA were weight less than 82 kg, minimal pain at rest, an arc of motion greater than 90°, flexion contracture less than 5°, and a passively correctable, angular deformity less than 15°.[23,24] Advances in surgical technique, implant design, and bearing surface technology[25] have contributed to expanded indications for UKA.

Younger, heavier, and more active patients undergoing UKA show excellent results.[26–35]

Early results of UKA in the ACL-deficient knee suggested aseptic loosening of the tibial component and greater eccentric prosthesis wear.[36,37] Goodfellow and colleagues reported a failure rate of 16.2% in the ACL-deficient mobile-bearing UKA,[37] whereas Deschamps and Lapeyre reported a failure rate of 87% in patients with at least 10 mm of preoperative anterior tibial translation on lateral weight-bearing radiograph at 7 years using a fixed-flat-bearing design with no keel.[36] In the mobile-bearing prosthesis, it is believed that ACL deficiency contributes to eccentric loading across the mobile-bearing polyethylene to the tibial base plate, contributing to failure and the need for revision surgery.[38]

More recent evidence suggests both fixed-bearing and mobile-bearing UKA with and without ACL reconstruction are viable options for the ACL-deficient, medial compartment arthritic knee. A revision rate of 1.2% was reported in 575 fixed-bearing UKAs in 415 patients at 9-year follow-up. Although the proportion of ACL-deficient knees was not reported, it was noted that the ACL was frequently absent with associated translatory deformity.[39] Another study of 10 ACL-deficient UKAs at an average of 12 years follow-up (range 10–18 years)[40] reported no patients required revision arthroplasty, 7 of 10 remained asymptomatic at the latest follow-up, 2 of 10 reported mild instability that did not interfere with activities, and 1 of 10 required a secondary ACL reconstruction for instability.

Technical factors such as proper tensioning of the collateral ligaments are key to successful outcomes, particularly in the ACL-deficient knee.[40] Changes in the posterior tibial slope contribute to tensioning of the collateral ligaments; an increase in the posterior tibial slope decreases collateral ligament tension and a decrease in the posterior tibial slope increases collateral ligament tension.[41–43] Fixed-bearing UKA in the ACL-deficient knee requires a smaller posterior tibial slope for a successful outcome. We recommend that the posterior tibial slope should be less than 7°.[41–43] A recent cadaveric model suggested that decreasing the posterior tibial slope of a medial UKA to approximately 4° significantly decreased anterior tibial translation during a Lachman maneuver in the ACL-deficient knee. Anterior tibial translation was not different from that of an ACL-intact knee after altering the posterior tibial slope.[25]

Osteophyte removal is another point of consideration when performing a UKA in the ACL-deficient knee. Osteophytes within the intercondylar notch may function as secondary static stabilizers of the knee.[40] Removal of these osteophytes and the ACL remnant/scar may contribute to postoperative instability. We have found that notch impingement from osteophytes must be dealt with for any successful UKA to attain good motion, but leaving all remnants of the ACL is essential to avoid destabilizing the knee.

The instability felt by a patient is typically not in the anteroposterior (AP) plane but rather in the medial-lateral plane. We believe that this instability is a result of medial collateral ligament shortening, which occurs preoperatively with the normal progression of OA. The direction of instability, if any, can be distinguished on careful history to help ensure a successful outcome in the ACL-deficient knee requiring a UKA. UKA remains an option in patients reporting medial-lateral instability during functional activities, whereas alternative treatment options should be explored in patients reporting AP instability.

Combined UKA and ACL Reconstruction

Another option for the ACL-deficient, arthritic knee is to reconstruct the ACL either before or at the time of the UKA. Early to midterm results are promising for both mobile-bearing and fixed-bearing prostheses.[44–48] Survivorship has been reported to be 93% at an average 5-year follow-up in 52 staged or simultaneous UKAs with ACL reconstruction[48] and 100% in 27 patients undergoing combined ACL-UKA reconstruction with evidence of improved knee stability.[46] Although these results are encouraging, more long-term outcomes studies are needed.

Concerns with a combined procedure include postoperative stiffness, improperly positioned ACL graft tunnels secondary to the prosthesis, graft impingement, undersizing of the tibial base plate to avoid graft impingement, the potential for a stress raiser or delayed proximal tibia fracture, and the risk of aseptic loosening of the tibial base plate, particularly in a mobile-bearing design if ACL reconstruction fails. As a result, staged reconstruction has been favored by our group. We have recently performed subchondroplasty for bony edema (insufficiency fractures) to avoid stress raisers and delayed fractures as well as to minimize the risk of aseptic loosening of the tibial component to ensure an excellent outcome.[49,50]

SELECTION CRITERIA
Patient Selection for UKA in the ACL-Deficient Patient

Patient selection is crucial for successful outcomes. Clinical decision making is challenging and should not be taken lightly by surgeon or patient alike.[51] Conservative treatment regimens should be exhausted before any surgical intervention. Although data may be lacking for the arthritic, ACL-deficient knee in the young, active individual, the surgeon can use the abundance of data in the younger, athletic ACL-deficient knee literature to guide operative treatment.[52]

The terminology of coper and noncoper emerged in the ACL literature to define the population of patients who have the ability to dynamically stabilize or cope with their knee disorder (eg, no instability events despite lacking a functional ACL).[53] In addition to the static, ligamentous stabilizers of the knee, dynamic stabilizers (eg, muscular contractions of the quadriceps, hamstrings and gastrocnemius muscles[54–56] and neuromuscular and proprioceptive physiologic responses[57–60]) contribute to knee stability during functional tasks. Studies have shown that high-level, ACL-deficient athletes without a reconstructed ACL perform similar to their peers who underwent ACL reconstruction at 10 years.[61] Likewise, many professional mogul skiers who have had an ACL reconstruction and overtime no longer have a functional ACL perform as well as their colleagues without a brace, performing to a level of excellence not fully understood.

Identification of ACL-Deficient Osteoarthritic Copers

A thorough history should always be conducted to identify knee instability. Specific questions without leading the patient should be asked by the surgeon. This process may take time but is worth the effort to manage expectations, leading to excellent long-term outcomes, in our opinion. The 1-finger test (ie, using 1 finger to point to the uncomfortable area) is used to determine the location of discomfort followed by a discussion about the noted instability (**Fig. 2**). It is important to decipher whether the instability is felt side to side or front to back. Almost all patients with an attritional tear of the ACL or chronic tear describe a side-to-side feeling of giving out. The description we use is "a knee falling into a pothole on the street." Most patients have a tight capsule because of the slow progression of their arthritis. Capsular contracture minimizes AP instability or giving way and can serve as a good indicator of patients who can have a successful UKA without an ACL reconstruction and return to a high level of activity. Reports of AP instability/subluxation events serve as a contraindication for UKA without reconstructing the ACL.

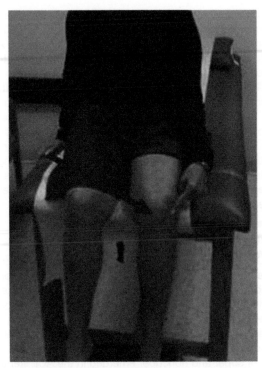

Fig. 2. The 1-finger test. On physical examination, the patient must point to the area of pain (*arrow*) with 1 finger to identify the area of discomfort.

Screening tools have been developed to identify copers from noncopers in the young, ACL-deficient, nonarthritic population.[62,63] A complete physical examination, including quadriceps strength testing, perturbation tolerance, timed, 6-meter single-leg hop test in the young athlete, and other plyometric testing, have been suggested as indicators of a person's ability to dynamically stabilize their knee when they have a compromised ACL.[51–57,61] Plyometric testing can be challenging in the older, arthritic population, because of pain and impact loading of the involved knee. Adaptations in the screening process can improve patient tolerance to testing and make the screening process more applicable to this patient subset with symptomatic OA. Because altered knee and gait biomechanics are well documented in the ACL-deficient patient population,[64,65] we suggest substituting single-leg hop testing with ambulation up and down stairs and a single limb step-down test to assess for instability with functional activities. Trampoline walking can also be used to ensure no frank instability. A common finding in this population is not a complaint of pain ascending stairs in the varus knee (pain ascending stairs is more commonly associated with the valgus knee) but rather more discomfort over the medial compartment descending stairs. Quadriceps and hamstring strength testing on an isokinetic dynamometer can also be performed; we recommend strength to be a minimum of 70% of the contralateral side.[66] For rare patients who would like to return to high-level, competitive singles tennis or soccer, we perform perturbation training and require no feeling of instability on a roller board or tilt board. We recommend a fixed-bearing UKA for this group of patients, whom we refer to as copers.

Additional criteria for considering a UKA for the ACL-deficient knee without concomitant ACL reconstruction include:

- Varus/valgus stability at 0° and 30° flexion with no more than 8-mm excursion and a firm end point
- Flexible varus deformity less than 15°, correctable to neutral with or without stress radiographs
- No tibial pseudosubluxation on an AP film of the knee (**Fig. 3**)
- Flexion range of motion of at least 105°
- A correctable flexion contracture of up to 5° is an acceptable finding with limited anterior subluxation of the tibia on the lateral extension radiographs

Noncopers are classified as having the following symptoms, no different from the copers as described earlier, with some exceptions. This group of patients do experience a giving way in the AP direction, much like a classic ACL-deficient patient describes. Their KT-1000 knee laxity testing device often shows greater than 10-mm side-to-side difference on manual maximum exertion. There are often episodes of giving out on a tilt board or any uneven ground testing. We recommend a staged procedure for these ACL-deficient, arthritic knees with an ACL reconstruction (bone-patellar tendon-bone allograft; graft donors always <40 years of age, because of the change in the collagen content) and a fixed-bearing prosthesis.

Contraindications to UKA in the ACL-deficient, arthritic knee are still those accepted by many when the patient has a fixed varus deformity (eg, not flexible on examination, not correctable to neutral on stress view radiograph). If the fixed varus deformity is greater than 8°, we do not offer an ACL reconstruction. If a UKA is performed in this subset of patients, the patient must understand they will continue to have a varus thrust yet no discomfort. If there is persistent anterior subluxation of the tibia, (>5 mm on a lateral weight-bearing radiograph), ACL reconstruction must be performed before a UKA. Patients with a fixed flexion contracture greater than 12° or a previous HTO, lateral compartment degenerative changes (Ahlback Stage 3 or higher)[67] and/or subluxation, and/or tricompartmental arthritis are all contraindicated for a UKA with an ACL reconstruction. All patients who undergo UKA with an ACL-deficient knee should

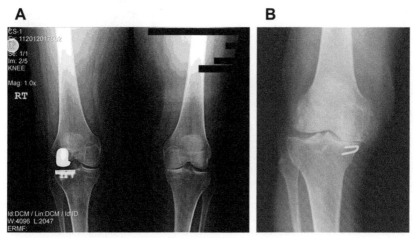

A   **B**

Fig. 3. (*A*) Preoperative radiograph (AP view) in an osteoarthritic ACL-deficient left knee. No evidence of tibial pseudosubluxation. (*B*) Evidence of pseudosubluxation.

expect pes bursitis, which typically resolves within 6 months. Pes bursitis in this population is treated conservatively and at times may require a steroid injection.

PREOPERATIVE PLANNING

It is hoped that setting preoperative guidelines has been reinforced in this article for successful outcomes. Education by the surgeon and health care provider (eg, nurse practitioner, physician assistant) should be provided pertaining to the risks, benefits, and alternative procedures so that patient and surgeon expectations are consistent. The patient's postoperative expectations are integral to the decision-making process in order to maximize long-term, postoperative outcomes with excellent patient satisfaction.[68]

SURGICAL PROCEDURE

The surgical approach we use, instrumentation use, and technique are explained in detail in the article on "Unicondylar Knee Arthroplasty: Intramedullary Technique" by Dunn and colleagues elsewhere in this issue. We use a fixed-bearing intramedullary technique with the distal femur cut first to be able to treat patients with flexion contractures preoperatively.

When a UKA is performed in the ACL-deficient knee, the intercondylar notch is carefully debrided of osteophytes in an effort to maintain stability (**Fig. 4**).[69,70] The fat pad is excised for visualization and to ensure that any restraint is removed for excellent patellar mobilization. The proximal tibial cut is set for 4-mm depth of resection, with a starting posterior tibial slope of 4°. If a solid anterior end point is not felt, the posterior tibial slope is then recut at 0° (**Fig. 5**). After insertion of trials, the knee is tensioned appropriately with a 2-mm tension gauge for a 9-mm or 10-mm polyethylene insert. The anterior drawer test is performed with the knee flexed to 90° and neutral rotation and the Lachman maneuver is performed in 30° of flexion. With proper patient

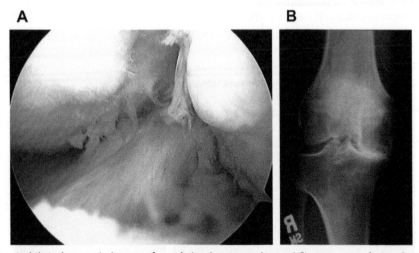

Fig. 4. (A) Arthroscopic image of notch impingement in an ACL-competent knee. Osteophytes are routinely removed to avoid notch impingement after placing a UKA. (B) AP plain radiograph in an ACL-deficient medial compartment osteoarthritic right knee with classic impingement. In ACL-deficient knees, the intercondylar notch is carefully debrided of osteophytes to maintain stability in the knee.

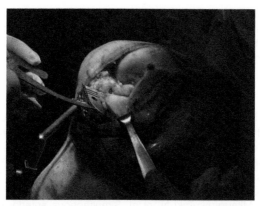

Fig. 5. Proximal tibial cut. The proximal tibial cut is initially set for 4-mm depth of resection and a starting posterior tibial slope of 4°.

selection, there is rarely a need to recut the tibia. The rest of the procedure is similar to an ACL-competent knee.

POSTOPERATIVE MANAGEMENT

Postoperative management is similar to reconstruction UKA. Although literature is lacking for the rehabilitation of patients with ACL-deficient UKA, intuitively, the incorporation of perturbation training, which has shown to be beneficial in rehabilitation protocols after ACL reconstruction, may be of great value and is certainly deserving of more research.[71] Our ACL rehabilitation is conservative and does not allow for any return to pivoting sports before 6 months. Patients undergoing UKA ACL-deficient or ACL-competent refrain from these activities for the same period.

OUTCOMES

Our review of the last 10 patients with ACL-deficient, arthritic knee performed by KDP has been promising. At the latest follow-up (mean 2.9 ± 3.0 years, range 1–8 years), patients with ACL-deficient UKA had similar outcomes to age, BMI, and gender-matched patients with UKA and competent ACL. Our patients with ACL-deficient knee and UKA have a Lysholm score of 92.4 ± 8.6, a Tegner score of 4.5 ± 2.0, a Hospital for Special Surgery score of 93.7 ± 7.6, a patient satisfaction score of 9.6 ± 0.82 (maximum score 10), knee flexion range of motion of 133° ± 11°, and knee extension range of motion 0°. Patients have returned to their previous recreational activities, including tennis and skiing.

SUMMARY

Management of the adult younger than 55 years and the physiologically mature adult with medial compartments arthritis and an ACL-deficient knee having failed conservative and simpler interventions remains a topic of debate and requires careful thought to manage. We have had success using our selection process. Our most common complication in the non-ACL reconstructed UKA is pes anserine bursitis. The bursitis typically emerges within the first 6 months postoperatively, typically at around 6 weeks, and is most likely related to increased pull from the hamstrings as a dynamic stabilizer in the now more mobile ACL-deficient knee. We have used classic, steroid injections for treatment of this event, with complete resolution in all patients by 6 months after UKA. Proper patient selection and education are the keys to success with this procedure. New surgical techniques have arisen that may prove to be successful over time; however, long-term follow-up (>15 years) is still required.

REFERENCES

1. Williams RJ III, Wickiewicz TL, Warren RF. Management of unicompartmental arthritis in the anterior cruciate ligament-deficient knee. Am J Sports Med 2000;28(5):749–60.
2. Noyes FR, Barber SD, Simon R. High tibial osteotomy and ligament reconstruction in varus angulated, anterior cruciate ligament-deficient knees. A two- to seven-year follow-up study. Am J Sports Med 1993;21(1):2–12.
3. Akamatsu Y, Mitsugi N, Taki N, et al. Simultaneous anterior cruciate ligament reconstruction and opening wedge high tibial osteotomy: Report of four cases. Knee 2010;17(2):114–8.
4. Machner A, Pap G, Krohn A, et al. Quadriceps muscle function after high tibial osteotomy for osteoarthritis of the knee. Clin Orthop Relat Res 2002;(399): 177–83.
5. Schallberger A, Jacobi M, Wahl P, et al. High tibial valgus osteotomy in unicompartmental medial osteoarthritis of the knee: A retrospective follow-up study over 13-21 years. Knee Surg Sports Traumatol Arthrosc 2011;19(1):122–7.
6. Brouwer RW, Bierma-Zeinstra SM, van Raaij TM, et al. Osteotomy for medial compartment arthritis of the knee using a closing wedge or an opening wedge controlled by a Puddu plate. A one-year randomised, controlled study. J Bone Joint Surg Br 2006;88(11):1454–9.
7. Sprenger TR, Doerzbacher JF. Tibial osteotomy for the treatment of varus gonarthrosis. Survival and failure analysis to twenty-two years. J Bone Joint Surg Am 2003;85(3):469–74.
8. Zaffagnini S, Bonanzinga T, Grassi A, et al. Combined ACL reconstruction and closing-wedge HTO for varus angulated ACL-deficient knees. Knee Surg Sports Traumatol Arthrosc 2013;21(4):934–41.
9. Graveleau N, DaSilva J, Litchfield R, et al. Clinical outcome after combined anterior cruciate ligament reconstruction and medial opening wedge high tibial osteotomy. J Bone Joint Surg Br 2008;90(Suppl I):109.
10. Bonnin MP, Salreta JF, Chambat P, et al. What can we really do following TKA, UKA and HTO? Arthroscopy 2012;28(9):e339–40.
11. Meding JB, Meding LK, Ritter MA, et al. Pain relief and functional improvement remain 20 years after knee arthroplasty. Clin Orthop Relat Res 2012;470(1):144–9.
12. Font-Rodriguez DE, Scuderi GR, Insall JN. Survivorship of cemented total knee arthroplasty. Clin Orthop Relat Res 1997;(345):79–86.
13. Alnahdi AH, Zeni JA, Snyder-Mackler L. Gait after unilateral total knee arthroplasty: frontal plane analysis. J Orthop Res 2011;29(5):647–52.
14. Yoshida Y, Mizner RL, Ramsey DK, et al. Examining outcomes from total knee arthroplasty and the relationship between quadriceps strength and knee function over time. Clin Biomech (Bristol, Avon) 2008;23(3):320–8.
15. Dennis DA, Komistek RD, Kim RH, et al. Gap balancing versus measured resection technique for total knee arthroplasty. Clin Orthop Relat Res 2010;468(1): 102–7.
16. Dennis DA, Komistek RD, Hoff WA, et al. In vivo knee kinematics derived using an inverse perspective technique. Clin Orthop Relat Res 1996;(331):107–17.

17. Stiehl JB, Dennis DA, Komistek RD, et al. In vivo determination of condylar lift-off and screw-home in a mobile-bearing total knee arthroplasty. J Arthroplasty 1999;14(3):293–9.
18. Stiehl JB, Komistek RD, Dennis DA, et al. Fluoroscopic analysis of kinematics after posterior-cruciate-retaining knee arthroplasty. J Bone Joint Surg Br 1995; 77(6):884–9.
19. Brugioni DJ, Andriacchi TP, Galante JO. A functional and radiographic analysis of the total condylar knee arthroplasty. J Arthroplasty 1990;5(2): 173–80.
20. Jones DL, Bhanegaonkar AJ, Billings AA, et al. Differences between actual and expected leisure activities after total knee arthroplasty for osteoarthritis. J Arthroplasty 2012;27(7):1289–96.
21. Lavernia CJ, Sierra RJ, Hungerford DS, et al. Activity level and wear in total knee arthroplasty: A study of autopsy retrieved specimens. J Arthroplasty 2001;16(4): 446–53.
22. Healy WL, Iorio R, Lemos MJ. Athletic activity after total knee arthroplasty. Clin Orthop Relat Res 2000;(380):65–71.
23. Kozinn SC, Scott R. Unicondylar knee arthroplasty. J Bone Joint Surg Am 1989; 71(1):145–50.
24. Borus T, Thornhill T. Unicompartmental knee arthroplasty. J Am Acad Orthop Surg 2008;16(1):9–18.
25. Oral E, Neils AL, Rowell SL, et al. Increasing irradiation temperature maximizes vitamin E grafting and wear resistance of ultrahigh molecular weight polyethylene. J Biomed Mater Res B Appl Biomater 2013;101(3):436–40.
26. Repicci JA, Hartman JF. Minimally invasive unicondylar knee arthroplasty for the treatment of unicompartmental osteoarthritis: An outpatient arthritic bypass procedure. Orthop Clin North Am 2004;35(2):201–16.
27. Price AJ, Waite JC, Svard U. Long-term clinical results of the medial Oxford unicompartmental knee arthroplasty. Clin Orthop Relat Res 2005;(435): 171–80.
28. Naudie D, Guerin J, Parker DA, et al. Medial unicompartmental knee arthroplasty with the Miller-Galante prosthesis. J Bone Joint Surg Am 2004;86(9): 1931–5.
29. Keblish PA, Briard JL. Mobile-bearing unicompartmental knee arthroplasty. A 2-center study with an 11-year (mean) follow-up. J Arthroplasty 2004;19(7 Suppl 2):87–94.
30. Berger RA, Meneghini RM, Jacobs JJ, et al. Results of unicompartmental knee arthroplasty at a minimum of ten years of follow-up. J Bone Joint Surg Am 2005; 87(5):999–1006.
31. Argenson JN, Chevrol-Benkeddache Y, Aubaniac JM. Modern unicompartmental knee arthroplasty with cement: A three to ten-year follow-up study. J Bone Joint Surg Am 2002;84(12):2235–9.
32. Swienckowski JJ, Pennington DW. Unicompartmental knee arthroplasty in patients sixty years of age or younger. J Bone Joint Surg Am 2004;86(Suppl 1 (Pt 2)):131–42.
33. Price AJ, Dodd CA, Svard UG, et al. Oxford medial unicompartmental knee arthroplasty in patients younger and older than 60 years of age. J Bone Joint Surg Br 2005;87(11):1488–92.
34. Pennington DW, Swienckowski JJ, Lutes WB, et al. Unicompartmental knee arthroplasty in patients sixty years of age or younger. J Bone Joint Surg Am 2003;85(10):1968–73.

35. Tabor OB Jr, Tabor OB, Bernard M, et al. Unicompartmental knee arthroplasty: long-term success in middle-age and obese patients. J Surg Orthop Adv 2005; 14(2):59–63.

36. Deschamps G, Lapeyre B. Rupture of the anterior cruciate ligament: A frequently unrecognized cause of failure of unicompartmental knee prostheses. Apropos of a series of 79 Lotus prostheses with a follow-up of more than 5 years. Rev Chir Orthop Reparatrice Appar Mot 1987;73(7):544–51 [in French].

37. Goodfellow JW, Kershaw CJ, Benson MK, et al. The Oxford knee for unicompartmental osteoarthritis. The first 103 cases. J Bone Joint Surg Br 1988;70(5): 692–701.

38. Goodfellow J, O'Connor J. The anterior cruciate ligament in knee arthroplasty. A risk-factor with unconstrained meniscal prostheses. Clin Orthop Relat Res 1992;(276):245–52.

39. Christensen NO. Unicompartmental prosthesis for gonarthrosis. A nine-year series of 575 knees from a Swedish hospital. Clin Orthop Relat Res 1991;(273): 165–9.

40. Cartier P, Sanouiller JL, Grelsamer RP. Unicompartmental knee arthroplasty surgery. 10-year minimum follow-up period. J Arthroplasty 1996;11(7):782–8.

41. Shao Q, MacLeod TD, Manal K, et al. Estimation of ligament loading and anterior tibial translation in healthy and ACL-deficient knees during gait and the influence of increasing tibial slope using EMG-driven approach. Ann Biomed Eng 2011;39(1):110–21.

42. Voos JE, Suero EM, Citak M, et al. Effect of tibial slope on the stability of the anterior cruciate ligament-deficient knee. Knee Surg Sports Traumatol Arthrosc 2012;20(8):1626–31.

43. Hernigou P, Deschamps G. Posterior slope of the tibial implant and the outcome of unicompartmental knee arthroplasty. J Bone Joint Surg Am 2004;86(3): 506–11.

44. Krishnan SR, Randle R. ACL reconstruction with unicondylar replacement in knee with functional instability and osteoarthritis. J Orthop Surg Res 2009;4:43.

45. Pandit H, Van Duren BH, Gallagher JA, et al. Combined anterior cruciate reconstruction and Oxford unicompartmental knee arthroplasty: In vivo kinematics. Knee 2008;15(2):101–6.

46. Tinius M, Hepp P, Becker R. Combined unicompartmental knee arthroplasty and anterior cruciate ligament reconstruction. Knee Surg Sports Traumatol Arthrosc 2012;20(1):81–7.

47. Pandit H, Beard DJ, Jenkins C, et al. Combined anterior cruciate reconstruction and Oxford unicompartmental knee arthroplasty. J Bone Joint Surg Br 2006; 88(7):887–92.

48. Weston-Simons JS, Pandit H, Jenkins C, et al. Outcome of combined unicompartmental knee replacement and combined or sequential anterior cruciate ligament reconstruction: A study of 52 cases with mean follow-up of five years. J Bone Joint Surg Br 2012;94(9):1216–20.

49. Sharkey PF, Cohen SB, Leinberry CF, et al. Subchondral bone marrow lesions associated with knee osteoarthritis. Am J Orthop 2012;41(9):413–7.

50. Roemer FW, Guermazi A, Javaid MK, et al. Change in MRI-detected subchondral bone marrow lesions is associated with cartilage loss: The MOST Study. A longitudinal multicentre study of knee osteoarthritis. Ann Rheum Dis 2009; 68(9):1461–5.

51. Sutton PM, Holloway ES. The young osteoarthritic knee: Dilemmas in management. BMC Med 2013;11:14.

52. Keyes GW, Carr AJ, Miller RK, et al. The radiographic classification of medial gonarthrosis. Correlation with operation methods in 200 knees. Acta Orthop Scand 1992;63(5):497–501.
53. Daniel DM, Stone ML, Dobson BE, et al. Fate of the ACL-injured patient. A prospective outcome study. Am J Sports Med 1994;22(5):632–44.
54. Andriacchi TP. Dynamics of pathological motion: Applied to the anterior cruciate deficient knee. J Biomech 1990;23(Suppl 1):99–105.
55. Limbird TJ, Shiavi R, Frazer M, et al. EMG profiles of knee joint musculature during walking: Changes induced by anterior cruciate ligament deficiency. J Orthop Res 1988;6(5):630–8.
56. Shiavi R, Zhang LQ, Limbird T, et al. Pattern analysis of electromyographic linear envelopes exhibited by subjects with uninjured and injured knees during free and fast speed walking. J Orthop Res 1992;10(2):226–36.
57. Wilk KE. Rehabilitation of isolated and combined posterior cruciate ligament injuries. Clin Sports Med 1994;13(3):649–77.
58. Johansson H, Sjolander P, Sojka P. Receptors in the knee joint ligaments and their role in the biomechanics of the joint. Crit Rev Biomed Eng 1991;18(5):341–68.
59. Johansson H. Role of knee ligaments in proprioception and regulation of muscle stiffness. J Electromyogr Kinesiol 1991;1(3):158–79.
60. Lephart SM, Pincivero DM, Giraldo JL, et al. The role of proprioception in the management and rehabilitation of athletic injuries. Am J Sports Med 1997;25(1):130–7.
61. Meuffels DE, Favejee MM, Vissers MM, et al. Ten year follow-up study comparing conservative versus operative treatment of anterior cruciate ligament ruptures. A matched-pair analysis of high level athletes. Br J Sports Med 2009;43(5):347–51.
62. Fitzgerald GK, Axe MJ, Snyder-Mackler L. A decision-making scheme for returning patients to high-level activity with nonoperative treatment after anterior cruciate ligament rupture. Knee Surg Sports Traumatol Arthrosc 2000;8(2):76–82.
63. Moksnes H, Snyder-Mackler L, Risberg MA. Individuals with an anterior cruciate ligament-deficient knee classified as noncopers may be candidates for nonsurgical rehabilitation. J Orthop Sports Phys Ther 2008;38(10):586–95.
64. Berchuck M, Andriacchi TP, Bach BR, et al. Gait adaptations by patients who have a deficient anterior cruciate ligament. J Bone Joint Surg Am 1990;72(6):871–7.
65. Andriacchi TP, Birac D. Functional testing in the anterior cruciate ligament-deficient knee. Clin Orthop Relat Res 1993;(288):40–7.
66. Taylor NA, Sanders RH, Howick EI, et al. Static and dynamic assessment of the Biodex dynamometer. Eur J Appl Physiol Occup Physiol 1991;62(3):180–8.
67. Ahlback S. Osteoarthrosis of the knee. A radiographic investigation. Acta Radiol Diagn (Stockh) 1968;(Suppl 277):7–72.
68. Greene KA, Harwin SF. Maximizing patient satisfaction and functional results after total knee arthroplasty. J Knee Surg 2011;24(1):19–24.
69. Hasegawa A, Otsuki S, Pauli C, et al. Anterior cruciate ligament changes in the human knee joint in aging and osteoarthritis. Arthritis Rheum 2012;64(3):696–704.
70. Wada M, Tatsuo H, Baba H, et al. Femoral intercondylar notch measurements in osteoarthritic knees. Rheumatology 1999;38(6):554–8.
71. Fitzgerald GK, Axe MJ, Snyder-Mackler L. The efficacy of perturbation training in nonoperative anterior cruciate ligament rehabilitation programs for physical active individuals. Phys Ther 2000;80(2):128–40.

UniCAP as an Alternative for Unicompartmental Arthritis

Anthony Miniaci, MD, FRCSC

KEYWORDS

- UniCAP • Medial tibiofemoral arthrosis • Joint surface mapping • Alternative

KEY POINTS

- Patient profiling is critical for successful individual care.
- Both tibial and femoral components should provide adequate defect coverage.
- Careful intra-operative mapping of the defect needs to be undertaken in order to match the prosthetic implant curvature to the curvature of the articular surface.
- A bony rim has to be maintained at the periphery of the tibial plateau to ensure bony stability.
- The cannulated system allows for perpendicular joint access; however, proper axis without excessive torque should be followed throughout implant bed preparation to avoid any pin or reamer deviation.
- Initial counter-clockwise rotation ensures an even cutting engagement into the tibial plateau.
- When placing the implant, carefully trim articular cartilage around the margin of implant. It is important to place each implant flush or recess slightly below the articular surface (0.5–1.0 mm) to avoid damage to the opposing articular surfaces.
- Uniform cement technique with pressurization should be achieved, especially surrounding the tibial component.

INTRODUCTION

In the past decade, the number of total knee arthroplasties (TKA) performed each year in the United States has doubled, with a disproportionate increase among adults between the ages of 45 and 64 years.[1] It is estimated that 4 million adults currently live with a total knee replacement; among those, 1.5 million are 50 to 69 years old.[1] Younger age, combined with longer life expectancy places a large number of patients at risk for complications or revisions. Wylde and colleagues[2] reported that up to 15% of total knee patients may encounter severe or extreme persistent pain 3 to 4 years after surgery.

Cleveland Clinic Lerner College of Medicine, Cleveland Clinic, 5555 Transportation Boulevard, Garfield Heights, OH 44125, USA
E-mail address: miniaca@ccf.org

Clin Sports Med 33 (2014) 57–65
http://dx.doi.org/10.1016/j.csm.2013.06.002
0278-5919/14/$ – see front matter © 2014 Elsevier Inc. All rights reserved.

sportsmed.theclinics.com

Based on these considerations, the full spectrum of focal, mono-and bicompartmental treatment options should be explored, especially in patients younger than 65 before total knee arthroplasty as an end-stage procedure is considered.

In the early stage of knee arthrosis, cartilage lesions frequently produce pain and functional limitations that are worse than those experienced with anterior cruciate ligament (ACL) deficiency and equal to those experienced by patients who are scheduled for knee arthroplasty.[3] In the younger population, this loss of quality of life relates to work-related deficits and higher socioeconomic costs.[3] Biological precursor treatments to arthroplasty aim at symptomatic pain relief and functional improvement, with emphasis on joint preservation returning the patient to his or her previous lifestyle while delaying or preventing the onset of osteoarthritis.[4–6]

Patients who find themselves between early and late-stage arthritis have been the target for less invasive arthroplasty procedures that maintain adequate bone stock and soft tissues to allow an uncomplicated exit into conventional joint replacement at a later stage. This transition from biology to arthroplasty has been less defined than early or late-stage procedures.

Given the premise of joint preservation, the first implant patients receive should be the least invasive to both bone and soft tissues. As such, the implant needs to be thin, contoured, and specific to the defect size and location in order to minimize the amounts of bone resected, so that future options such as knee arthroplasty are not compromised. To address these goals, a novel knee resurfacing technology was introduced over the past decade facilitating knee surface reconstruction. with more than 70 implant sizes and shapes (Arthrosurface, Inc., Franklin, Massachusetts). The platform consists of intraoperative surface measurement and placement of a defect-sized implant into the native joint surface. Compared with conventional arthroplasty, metallic resurfacing utilizes inlay prosthetic placement that preserves healthy surrounding tissues. In contrast to unicondylar knee replacement (UKA), tibiofemoral knee resurfacing (UniCAP, Arthrosurface, Inc.) allows for a meniscal sparing procedure. The modular system not only places emphasis on individual fit, but also requires proper disease staging and patient selection in order to maximize individual success.

PATIENT SELECTION

Patient profiling through detailed pre- and intraoperative assessment ensures individual patient care and optimized outcomes. The ideal candidate is typically between 40 and 60 years of age, has failed previous conservative treatment and biologic procedures, and presents with focal but bipolar tibiofemoral arthrosis.

Preoperative physical and radiological examinations should show a range of motion deficit of less than 10° flexion or 5° of extension, and no mechanical malalignment greater than 5°. It is unknown whether the meniscus needs to be intact for this procedure to be successful, but one would presume that having some meniscal function would lead to better results. Meniscal extrusion and loss of more than 50% of the meniscus suggest a more advanced process and would be of concern. The knee should not show any evidence of bony deformities, erosions, or cystic formations, as inlay resurfacing cannot address bone loss. Standard anteroposterior (AP) and lateral radiographs and the Rosenberg 45° standing posteroanterior (PA) view aid in tibiofemoral staging, The Merchant view provides valuable information on the state of the patellofemoral joint. Preoperative magnetic resonance imaging (MRI) establishes further details on joint status and the tibiofemoral arthrosis and status of the patellofemoral joint. Both femoral and tibial defects should be effectively covered by the resurfacing components, but sometimes this is not possible. It is still unclear as to how much of the focal defect needs to be covered to achieve a successful result, but the author strives for full coverage if possible. This is reconfirmed intraoperatively. Secondary defects in other compartments should be evaluated and attended to, as they may be a source of symptoms. A combination of medial and patellofemoral pathology is common and may need to be addressed.

The expectations of the patient and physical demands to be placed on the knee have to be taken into consideration. Risk factors such as high body mass index (BMI), meniscal insufficiency, ligament laxity, mechanical alignment, metabolic disorders affecting bone quality, and concomitant cartilage deficits outside the coverage area have to be carefully assessed, and compounding effects of comorbidities need to be considered when establishing a treatment plan.

PROSTHETIC DESIGN

The femoral articulating component (CoCrMo) is available in 2 sizes (27 or 40 mm diameter) and a variety of surface convexities that match the intraoperative surface measurements at the defect site. Implant stability is facilitated through a shallow bone bed, tapered screw (Ti), and secondary osteo-integration with the undersurface coating (Ti) (**Fig. 1**). The 20 mm tibial component (UHMWPE) is cemented into a tibial implant bed.

SURGICAL TECHNIQUE (MEDIAL COMPARTMENT)
Arthroscopic Focal Tibial Resurfacing

The patient is placed and draped for standard knee arthroscopy, allowing high knee flexion on the table. A full-length skin incision is performed prior to arthroscopy to facilitate tissue dissection and avoid challenges caused by fluid extravasations during arthroscopy. The incision is extended beyond the distal joint line to improve exposure and avoid interference during the femoral preparation. Throughout the arthroscopic tibial preparation, capsular integrity is maintained by limiting the capsulotomy to the antero-medial portal.

Following arthroscopic exploration and concurrent treatment as indicated, 2 contact probes can be used to confirm adequate defect coverage on the femoral

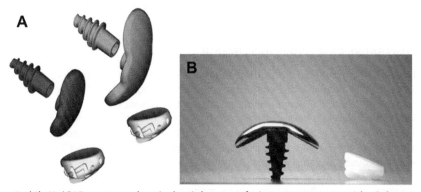

Fig. 1. (A) UniCAP contoured articular inlay resurfacing components with defect-sized femoral and tibial components. (B) Engaged morse taper connection combining the articular and fixation components on the femoral condyle (40 mm diameter) (left). Profile view of the all-polyethylene (UHMWPE) tibial component (20 mm).

side before arthroscopic-assisted tibial resurfacing is carried out. Because of the tibial roll back during physiological knee flexion, arthroscopic visualization offers inherent advantages for tibial preparation and implant placement. The knee is flexed to 20° to 30° under valgus stress, and tibial templates reconfirm defect coverage, surface fit, and establish a working axis for preparation of the tibial implant bed. Similar to ACL tibial tunnel preparation, a guide pin is placed from the antero-medial tibia through the center of the template. A cannulated pilot drill follows the guide pin to establish the tibial tunnel. A set of tibial tunnel instruments pre-pares for stop-controlled retrograde preparation of the tibial implant bed. Once reamed to the appropriate depth, a sizing trial is used to ensure slightly recessed implant margins. Prior to placement of the final tibial component, the femoral side is prepared.

Femoral Resurfacing

Following the conclusion of the arthroscopic procedure, the capsulotomy is expanded to expose the defect on the distal femoral condyle. With the knee in 90° to 120° of flexion, a femoral drill guide is placed over the defect with 4 points of contact to estab-lish a perpendicular working axis that is maintained through stepwise use of a guide pin, centering shaft, and medial/lateral and anterior/posterior contact probes measuring the individual joint surface curvature at the defect site. More flexion allows for posterior placement of the femoral implant. Treatment is individualized for each pa-tient, so that the implant is placed over the damaged area. A guide block is attached to provide perpendicular and depth-controlled surface reaming of the femoral implant bed. Once slightly recessed margins have been confirmed, the fixation screw is advanced into the center of the implant bed.

Attention is returned to implant the final tibial component using retrograde cement injection with pressurization against downward suture pull through the tibial tunnel, providing an even cement column around and underneath the tibial inlay. Proper cement fill is achieved when a uniform cement film has covered the intra-articular implant margins. A small curette is used to clean the component edges.

A small amount of cement is applied to the underside of the femoral component so as to not interfere with the taper connection. The implant is then impacted, engaging the morse taper connection with the screw. This small amount of cement does not appear to interfere with any revision efforts that may be necessary in the future.

The joint is thoroughly lavaged, and the capsulotomy and skin incision are closed according to standard practice.

POSTOPERATIVE CARE AND REHABILITATION

Following the procedure, cold compresses have shown to reduce analgesics and improve quality of life in the early postoperative period along with decreasing the amount of swelling.[7–9] Weight bearing as tolerated is encouraged for 2 to 6 weeks while slowly weaning patients off their crutches. Home or formal physical therapy ex-ercises are encouraged, and range-of-motion exercises are started immediately. Strengthening can begin as soon as pain and swelling have reduced to acceptable levels. However, patients should not return to sporting activity or other high-demand activities until full range of motion is achieved with no pain or swelling present. There appears to be a 2-tage recovery for many of these patients. Initial postoperative recovery of motion and ambulation occurs very quickly, with most achieving excellent range in the first 3 to 6 weeks. Very active patients sometimes can have ongoing symptoms, especially with high-load activities that can improve after 6 to 9 months.

Patience and full strength and adherence to a good rehabilitation protocol are optimal for a successful recovery.

RESULTS

Thirty-eight knees in 35 patients with a mean age of 48.3 years (range 23–80 years) were treated with tibiofemoral resurfacing.[10] Prior procedures included 27 meniscectomies, 14 microfractures, 4 ACL reconstructions, 3 mosaicplasties, 2 osteotomies and 2 refixations of osteochondral defects. The Kellgren Lawrence osteoarthritis grade for the medial femoral condyle (MFC) was 3.95 (range 3–4), and the medial tibial plateau (MTP) was 3.86 (range 2–4). The average Outerbridge classification for the MFC and the MTP was 2.94 (**Table 1**). There were 18 concomitant partial meniscectomies conducted, 3 ACL reconstructions, and 1 high tibial osteotomy. Medial and trochlear resurfacing occurred in 8 cases.

At an average follow-up of 18.7 months (range 12–27 months), statistically significant improvement in Knee Injury and Osteoarthritis Outcome Score (KOOS) scores was achieved in the subdomains of pain, symptoms, activities and sports (**Table 2**). Pain VAS went from 6.9 at baseline to 2.7 at follow-up, and normal range of motion was achieved in 89% of the cases within 6 weeks of the surgery. No implant subsidence, disengagement, or periprosthetic cyst formation was observed. A significant improvement in physical function and bodily pain subscales of the SF-12 were observed, and this improvement reconfirmed the results of the KOOS domains (**Table 3**).

DISCUSSION

The author's experience with tibiofemoral resurfacing demonstrates significant clinical improvement across meaningful endpoints of the cartilage repair validated KOOS score.[11,12]

In light of the high incidence of failed cartilage precursor treatments, tibiofemoral resurfacing not only maintained bone, articular cartilage, and meniscal function, but also performed well in concomitant ACL reconstruction (**Fig. 2**) and high tibial osteotomy when indicated. The modular system not only places emphasis on individual fit, but at the same time requires proper disease staging and patient selection in order to maximize individual success. In such, limited resurfacing is less forgiving than more invasive procedures that sacrifice surface beyond the pathological margins.

Individual patient care in the long-term management of knee arthritis is essential to not only improve patient outcomes, satisfaction, return to work, and activities, but also to reduce the burden of TKA for a relatively young patient population. Maximizing

Table 1 Preoperative staging		
Location	**Kellgren Lawrence OA Grade**	**Outerbridge Classification**
Medial femoral condyle	3.95 (range 3–4)	2.94
Medial tibial plateau	3.86 (range 2–4)	2.94
Trochlea	2.24 (range 0–4)	1.26
Patella	1.87 (range 0–3)	1.26
Lateral femoral condyle	1.43 (range 0–3)	1.0
Lateral tibial plateau	1.47 (range 0–3)	1.0

Table 2
KOOS domain scores

Domain	Preoperative	Postoperative	P Value
Pain	48.42	72.24	<.001*
Symptoms	45.71	69.98	<.001*
Activity	55.27	80.62	<.001*
Sports	19.9	43.04	<.001*
Quality of life	31.25	47.48	.07

* P<.05.

biologic precursor procedures and utilizing patient- and defect-specific resurfacing implants as a first line of implants when transition into arthroplasty becomes necessary, all help to delay TKA and reduce the risk of early revision. Because of the inherent inlay design, UniCAP knee resurfacing is not a replacement for UKA, but an early treatment alternative to bipolar knee arthrosis of the medial compartment in patients with otherwise healthy articular surfaces. Its clinical benefits are maximized if adequate defect coverage is afforded by both components, and the femoro-tibial compartment does not show any signs of bone loss; additionally, the patient should maintain more than 50% of meniscal function, and have less than 5° of malalignment and display a ligamentously stable knee. BMI of less than 30 kg/m² to avoid excessive loading of knee is ideal. A preoperative weight loss program can significantly add to the postoperative benefit: every 1 pound reduction in body weight reduces the overall force across the knee in a single leg stance by 2 to 3 pounds.[13,14]

Historically, UKA has achieved very satisfactory results, and implant registries have reported a 10-year success rate of 73% to 81%.[15,16] UKA provides benefits over TKA in the form of better knee kinematics, faster recovery, less trauma to tissues, and preservation of bone stock. It also allows for the conversion to a total knee if needed for disease progression.[17] UKA in the younger patient population (<60 years) has been shown to lower implant survival with increased revision rates. Kuipers[18] found an adjusted 2.2-fold increased risk of revision in this age group when compared to those older than 60 years. His cumulated survival rate at 5 years was 77.2% in younger patients, which increased to 89.4% in older patients (>60 years). Others have suggested that the lower survival rate is caused by a more active and demanding lifestyle, together with higher preoperative expectations of younger patients.[15,19] Increased polyethylene wear was found in patients younger than 55 years in a study by Felts.[20] When compared with TKA, UKA has also shown a higher revision

Table 3
SF-12 subdomain scores

Domain	Preoperative	Postoperative	P Value
PCS	37.34	43.48	.07
MCS	55.07	53.03	.40
Physical function	36.62	43.43	.04*
Role function	40.16	45.49	.10
Bodily Pain	35.56	43.50	.03*

* P<.05.

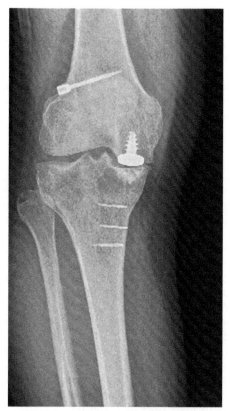

Fig. 2. Postoperative AP radiograph following tibiofemoral UniCAP resurfacing and concomitant ACL reconstruction.

rate;[21,22] therefore. caution should be used when suggesting UKA in the younger population,[23] as many have considered young age to be a contraindication for this procedure.[19,24–27]

Older patients with advanced stages of mono, bi- or tricompartment arthrosis have shown long-term survivorship of UKA and TKA; however, these designs are less amenable for early prosthetic intervention in limited bipolar, mono-compartmental lesions in middle-aged patients. Bourne and colleagues[28] reported that only 19% of patients were satisfied with the outcome of their total knee replacement. One of the big factors in the patient dissatisfaction for TKA was hospital in-patient treatment. As an alternative, UniCAP resurfacing can be completed on an out-patient basis, with accelerated recovery from surgery. Using this less invasive option, younger patients (<45 years) with bifocal knee arthrosis are returned to work and activities with pain relief and improved function before possibly having to undergo a TKA.

SUMMARY

The introduction of small knee implants over the past decade has stimulated discussion on the continuum of care for knee arthrosis and arthritis. Patient treatment has been afforded a new reconstructive layer with the goal of delaying end-stage arthroplasty procedure until later in life. The modular system is part of a joint preservation initiative with its origin in biologic precursor treatments addressing only disease-specific areas while maintaining healthy articular structures. As with focal biologic treatments, tibiofemoral resurfacing affords and requires individual profiling and patient counseling to address long-term management of knee arthritis.

UniCAP resurfacing is a promising new treatment option, although larger patient series are needed to further substantiate patient selection criteria and clinical performance. As the appropriate indications for this procedure continue to be defined, long term follow-up data will be reported.

REFERENCES

1. Weinstein AM, Rome BN, Reichmann WM, et al. Estimating the burden of total knee replacement in the United States. J Bone Joint Surg Am 2013;95:1–8.
2. Wylde V, Hewlett S, Learmonth ID, et al. Persistent pain after joint replacement: prevalence, sensory qualities, and postoperative determinants. Pain 2011; 152(3):566–72.
3. Heir S, Nerhus TK, Røtterud JH, et al. Focal cartilage defects in the knee impair quality of life as much as severe osteoarthritis a comparison of knee injury and osteoarthritis outcome score in 4 patient categories scheduled for knee surgery. Am J Sports Med 2010;38(2):231–7.
4. Cole BJ, Farr J, Winalski CS, et al. Outcomes after a single-stage procedure for cell-based cartilage repair: a prospective clinical safety trial with 2-year follow-up. Am J Sports Med 2011;39(6):1170–9.
5. Hjelle K, Solheim E, Strand T, et al. Articular cartilage defects in 1000 knee arthroscopies. Arthroscopy 2002;18(7):730–4.
6. Maletius W, Messner K. The effect of partial meniscectomy on the long-term prognosis of knees with localized, severe chondral damage. A twelve- to fifteen-year followup. Am J Sports Med 1996;24(3):258–62.
7. Schroder D, Passler HH. Combination of cold and compression after knee surgery. Knee Surg Sports Traumatol Arthrosc 1994;93:1–8.
8. Whitelaw GP, DeMuth KA, Demos HA, et al. The use of the Cryo/Cuff versus ice and elastic wrap in the postoperative care of knee arthroscopy patients. Am J Knee Surg 1995;8(1):28–30.
9. Woolf SK, Barfield WR, Merrill KD, et al. Comparison of a continuous temperature-controlled cryotherapy device to a simple icing regimen following outpatient knee arthroscopy. J Knee Surg 2008;21(1):15–9.
10. Miniaci A, Arneja S, Jones M. Clinical results of a novel knee resurfacing arthroplasty for focal osteoarthritis of the knee. ISAKOS; 2011.
11. Engelhart L, Nelson L, Lewis S, et al. Validation of the knee injury and osteoarthritis outcome score subscales for patients with articular cartilage lesions of the knee. Am J Sports Med 2012;40(10):2264–72.
12. Bekkers JE, de Windt TS, Raijmakers NJ, et al. Validation of the Knee Injury and Osteoarthritis Outcome Score (KOOS) for the treatment of focal cartilage lesions. Osteoarthr Cartil 2009;17(11):1434–9.
13. Felson DT, Lawrence RC, Dieppe PA, et al. Osteoarthritis: new insights. Part 1: the disease and its risk factors. Ann Intern Med 2000;133:635–46.
14. Ding C, Cicuttini F, Scott F, et al. Knee structural alteration and BMI: a cross-sectional study. Obes Res 2005;13(2):350–61.
15. Furnes O, Espehaug B, Lie SA, et al. Failure mechanisms after unicompartmental and tricompartmental primary knee replacement with cement. J Bone Joint Surg Am 2007;89(3):519–25.

16. Koskinen E, Paavolainen P, Eskelinen A, et al. Unicondylar knee replacement for primary osteoarthritis: a prospective follow-up study of 1819 patients from the Finnish arthroplasty register. Acta Orthop 2007;78(1):128–35.
17. Laurencin CT, Zelicof SB, Scott RD, et al. Unicompartmental versus total knee arthroplasty in the same patient. A comparative study. Clin Orthop Relat Res 1991; 273:151–6.
18. Kuipers BM, Kollen BJ, Kaijser Bots PC, et al. Factors associated with reduced early survival in the Oxford phase III medial compartment knee replacement. The Knee 2010;17:48–52.
19. Price AJ, Dodd CA, Svard UG, et al. Oxford medial unicompartmental knee arthroplasty in patients younger and older than 60 years of age. J Bone Joint Surg Br 2005;87(11):1488–92.
20. Felts E, Parratte S, Pauly V, et al. Function and quality of life following medial unicompartmental knee arthroplasty in patients 60 years of age or younger. Orthop Traumatol Surg Res 2010;96:861–7.
21. Gioe TJ, Novak C, Sinner P, et al. Knee arthroplasty in the young patient. Clin Orthop Relat Res 2007;464:83–7.
22. W-Dahl A, Robertsson O, Lidgren L. Surgery for knee osteoarthritis in younger patient. A Swedish register study. Acta Orthop 2010;81:161–4.
23. Pagnano MW, Clarke HD, Jacofsky DJ, et al. Surgical treatment of the middle-aged patient with arthritic knees. Instr Course Lect 2005;54:251–9.
24. Deshmukh RV, Scott RD. Unicompartmental knee arthroplasty for younger patients. Clin Orthop Relat Res 2002;44:108–22.
25. Schai PA, Suh J, Thornhill TS, et al. Unicompartmental knee arthroplasty in middle-aged patients: a 2- to 6-year follow-up evaluation. J Arthroplasty 1998; 13:365–72.
26. Engh GA, McAuley JP. Unicondylar arthroplasty: an option for high-demand patients with gonarthrosis. Instr Course Lect 1999;48:143–8.
27. Kozinn SC, Scott R. Unicondylar knee arthroplasty. J Bone Joint Surg Am 1989; 71:145–50.
28. Bourne RB, Chesworth BM, Davis AM, et al. Patient Satisfaction after total knee arthroplasty. Who is satisfied, and who is not? Clin Orthop Relat Res 2010;468: 57–63.

Unicondylar Knee
The Arthrex Experience

Alan Valadie, MD

KEYWORDS

- Unicondylar knee • Unicompartmental knee • Gap balancing • Kinematics

KEY POINTS

- Gap balancing in unicondylar knee arthroplasty is important to optimize range of motion and stability.
- A gap balancing system allows the surgeon to adjust bony resection levels to achieve symmetric flexion and extension gaps.
- A common scenario in the medial unicondylar knee is an extension space that is larger than the flexion space due to distal bone and cartilage loss. This can be managed by decreasing the distal femoral resection by the difference in the gaps.
- A gap balanced unicondylar knee arthroplasty system can result in kinematics similar to a normal knee.

INTRODUCTION

The ideal joint arthroplasty is one that maintains normal joint kinematics and proprioception, thereby optimizing function and contributing to a more normal "feel" of the knee. Unicondylar knee arthroplasty (UKA) is well suited to fulfill this goal, having been shown to replicate normal knee kinematics more than total knee arthroplasty.[1] This replication has been confirmed using gait analysis of both medial and lateral compartment UKA.[2] Maintenance of the cruciate ligaments and most of the normal anatomic structures of the knee are critical factors in this regard.

One feature common to both UKA and total knee arthroplasty is the concept of balanced flexion and extension gaps, which allows collateral ligament isometry as the knee moves from flexion to extension and maintains joint stability throughout range of motion. In UKA, gap balancing coupled with joint line restoration should lead to fairly normal knee kinematics.

If gaps are not balanced during the procedure, there will likely be effects on range of motion and/or stability. For example, if the final extension gap is larger than the flexion gap, there are 2 potential results: the knee will be stable in extension but tight in flexion, limiting knee range of motion, or the knee will be balanced in flexion but loose and unstable in extension.

Coastal Orthopedics and Sports Medicine, Bradenton, Florida 34209, USA
E-mail address: alanv@coastalorthopedics.com

Clin Sports Med 33 (2014) 67–76
http://dx.doi.org/10.1016/j.csm.2013.08.005
0278-5919/14/$ – see front matter © 2014 Elsevier Inc. All rights reserved.

Appropriate patient selection helps maximize the chances of reproducing normal kinematics. Although indications for UKA have expanded, avoiding UKA in patients with certain problems such as anterior cruciate ligament deficiency or significant deformity requiring substantial ligament releases is important. Engh and Ammeen[3] showed sliding motion in an anterior cruciate ligament–deficient knee accelerates polyethylene wear in UKA.

TECHNIQUE

The surgical procedure starts with the approach, minimizing ligament releases. An excessive medial release can result in the need to overcorrect the varus knee into valgus to obtain appropriate ligament tension. Overcorrecting knee alignment into valgus has been shown to accelerate cartilage wear in the lateral compartment and adversely affect survivorship.[4]

Bony preparation starts with the osteophyte removal followed by tibial resection, matching the native tibial slope. In a normal knee, the tibia rotates with flexion and extension around a fixed axis.[5] Making this tibial cut first creates a reference point in flexion and extension that helps determine proper anatomic positioning of the femoral component. It is important to remember that the tibial cut is the basis for the remainder of the bone preparation, so it is critical that this cut be perpendicular to the long axis of the tibia in the coronal plane.

Once the tibial cut is made, flexion and extension gaps are assessed with the use of spacer blocks (**Fig. 1**). Spacer blocks accomplished 2 main functions: first, they assess the thickness of the polyethylene and ensure adequate tibial resection. Second, they assess any potential differences between extension and flexion gaps.

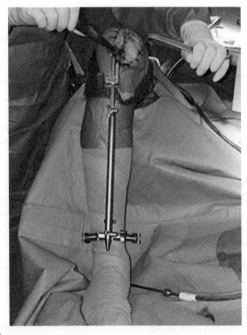

Fig. 1. Tibial resection.

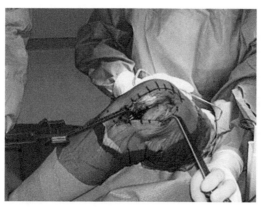

Fig. 2. Flexion gap.

Decisions can be made about bone resections based on findings with the gap analysis (**Figs. 2** and **3**). If the spacer block matching the minimum composite tibial thickness (8 mm in the Arthrex system) will not fit, then the tibial resection is too conservative and the components simply will not fit without overtightening the medial collateral ligament or performing ligament releases. In this scenario more tibial bone should be resected.

If a spacer block fits in both flexion and extension with appropriate slight ligament laxity (1 mm of laxity), then bone resections of the distal and posterior femur should be identical and equal to the thickness of the femoral component, which is typical in the knee without bony defects. Under these circumstances, if an 8-mm spacer block fits appropriately, it will likely be that an 8-mm-thick polyethylene will be the appropriate implant. If a 10-mm block fits symmetrically, the final tibial insert will likely be 10 mm.

A common scenario in the medially arthritic knee is for the extension gap to be larger than the flexion gap, typically the result of distal bone and cartilage loss. The posterior medial femoral condylar bone, and often the articular cartilage, may be preserved in medial compartment arthritis. In this setting, it takes a larger spacer block to fill the extension gap than it takes to fill the flexion gap. As an example, if the flexion gap is 8 mm and the extension gap is 10 mm, then the joint line should be moved distantly

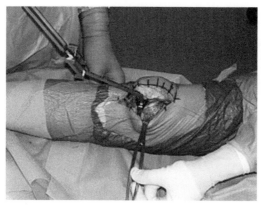

Fig. 3. Extension gap.

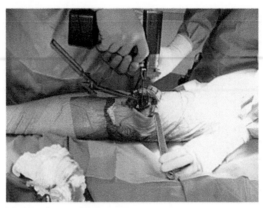

Fig. 4. Linked distal femoral resection.

2 mm by decreasing the depth of femoral resection. If the difference in flexion and extension gaps is 1 mm, then 1 mm less bone should be resected distally. This difference allows the surgeon to equalize the flexion and extension gaps. The ideal UKA instrument system allows such customization of the resection depth both distally and posteriorly (**Fig. 4**).

Once distal and posterior femoral resections have been made, the gaps can be rechecked to ensure they are symmetric. The gaps at this stage should equal the thickness of the femoral component plus the composite tibial thickness with 1 mm of additional laxity to avoid excess ligament tension. In the Arthrex system with an 8-mm tibial insert, this overall gap thickness would be 16 mm (7-mm femoral component thickness plus 8-mm tibial thickness plus 1-mm laxity) (**Figs. 5** and **6**).

Once the gaps are balanced and the joint line is re-established, then the distal femoral and proximal tibial preparations are completed. A trial reduction is carried out to confirm proper alignment, ligament tension, and range of motion. Final components are then implanted.

LEARNING CURVE

The learning curve for a gap balancing approach to UKA involves the following steps: (1) familiarization with the concept of balanced flexion and extension gaps;

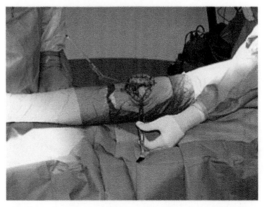

Fig. 5. Extension gap.

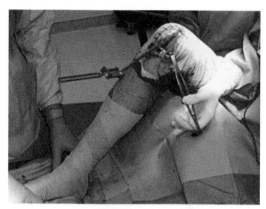

Fig. 6. Flexion gap.

(2) utilization of spacer blocks following tibial resection to assess the flexion and extension gaps and any potential differences between the two; (3) adjustment of femoral bony resection levels, which depends on the results of the gap analysis.

The Arthrex system allows these steps with a simple-to-use, streamlined system. It is also amenable for use in lateral compartment UKA.

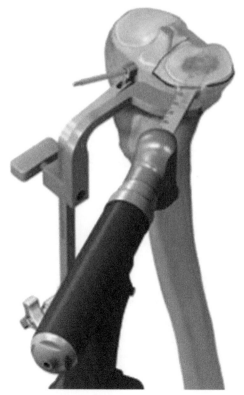

Fig. 7. Tibial resection.

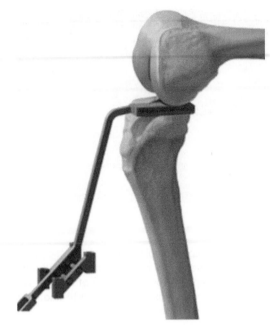

Fig. 8. Flexion gap.

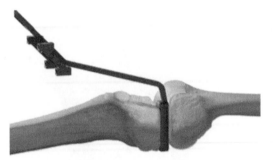

Fig. 9. Extension gap.

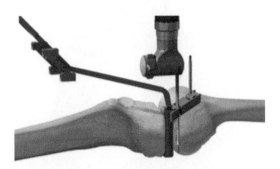

Fig. 10. Linked distal femoral resection.

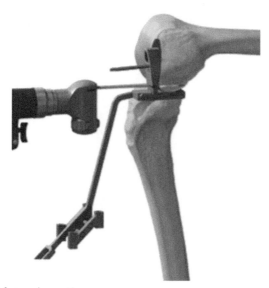

Fig. 11. Posterior femoral resection.

INSTRUMENTATION

The technique of UKA with the Arthrex system steps are as follows:

1. Exposure
2. Tibial resection
3. Gap analysis
4. Linked distal femoral resection
5. Posterior femoral resection
6. Final gap analysis (**Figs. 7–12**)
7. Completion of femoral preparation
8. Trial
9. Completion of tibial preparation
10. Final component implantation (**Figs. 13–16**)

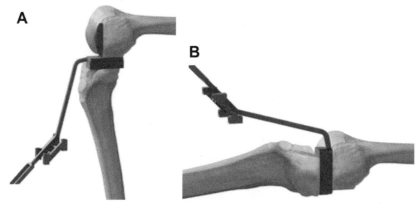

Fig. 12. Final gap analysis.

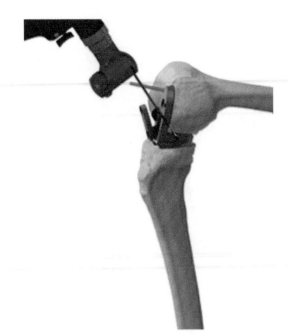

Fig. 13. Completion of femoral preparation.

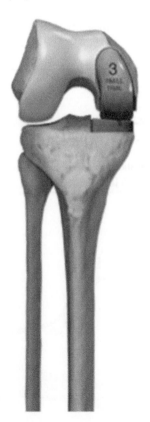

Fig. 14. Trial.

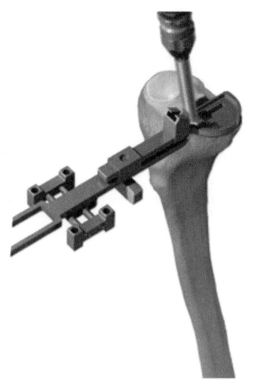

Fig. 15. Completion of tibial preparation.

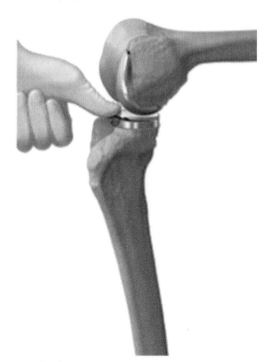

Fig. 16. Final component implantation.

REFERENCES

1. Patil S, Colwell CW, Ezzet KA, et al. Can normal knee kinematics be restored with unicompartmental arthroplasty. J Bone Joint Surg Am 2005;87(2):332–8. http://dx.doi.org/10.2106/JBJS.C.01467.
2. Fu YC, Simpson KJ, Kinsey TL, et al. Does interlimb knee symmetry exist after unicompartmental arthroplasty of the knee. Presented at the Annual meeting of the Knee Society. Clin Orthop Relat Res 2013;47(1):142–9.
3. Engh GA, Ammeen D. Is an intact anterior cruciate ligament needed in order to have a well-functioning unicondylar knee replacement? Clin Orthop Relat Res 2004;(428):170–3.
4. Henigou P, Deschamps G. Alignment influences wear in the knee after unicompartmental arthroplasty. Clin Orthop Relat Res 2004;423:161–5.
5. Eckhoff D, Hogan C, DiMatteo L, et al. Difference between the epicondylar and cylindrical axis of the knee. Clin Orthop Relat Res 2007;461:238–44.

The Simple Unicondylar Knee
Extramedullary Technique

Brett Levine, MD, MS, Aaron G. Rosenberg, MD*

KEYWORDS

- Unicompartmental • Extramedullary guides • Spacer blocks

KEY POINTS

- Extramedullary (EM) options exist for the surgical technique of unicompartmental knee arthroplasty (UKA) and include true EM and spacer block techniques.
- EM instrumentation relies on linked resection guides based on parallel cuts on the tibia and femur in setting the resection space, which accounts for the thickness of the implanted components.
- EM and spacer block techniques eliminate the need for cannulating the femur and the associated risks of marrow emboli. Postsurgical blood loss from the medullary canal may be reduced in these cases as well.
- Slight undercorrection or neutral alignment is favored with this technique and markers may be placed during surgery (under fluoroscopy) at the center of the ankle and hip to guide alignment rods.
- The EM technique dictates that the distal femoral resection level and targeting guide be pinned in place with the deformity being manually corrected and held in this position while securing the cutting blocks.
- Caution should be taken with a flexion contracture greater than 5° because it may be unsuccessful, and intramedullary technique should be considered.
- Alternative techniques should be considered with a knee that has a deformity that cannot be passively corrected.

INTRODUCTION

Recent reports have described 10-year survivorship of unicompartmental knee arthroplasty (UKA) ranging from 80.2% to 98%.[1–4] In order to maintain this high level of success it is important to follow meticulous surgical technique as well as stringent patient indications. Although UKA has long been popular in European countries, it is only recently that there has been a resurgence of partial knee replacements in the United States, predominantly fueled by patient demands, reliable instrumentation, and improved surgical techniques.[5] Several options exist regarding instrumentation for

Rush University Medical Center, Chicago, IL 60612, USA
* Corresponding author.
E-mail address: aarongbone@gmail.com

Clin Sports Med 33 (2014) 77–85
http://dx.doi.org/10.1016/j.csm.2013.06.003
0278-5919/14/$ – see front matter © 2014 Elsevier Inc. All rights reserved.

UKA, including intramedullary (IM), spacer block, and extramedullary (EM) techniques. A uniform theme regardless of the surgical technique is to err on the side of restoring a neutral mechanical axis or undercorrection of the deformity, so as not to incite degeneration of remaining the native compartments.[6] When performed appropriately, each of the surgical measures provides successful and reproducible results. This article focuses on the simple techniques of using the EM and spacer block guides for performing a UKA.

INDICATIONS

Among the most important factors in generating successful outcomes after UKA is identifying and selecting the appropriate surgical candidates. Such criteria include isolated clinical and radiographic findings in 1 compartment of the affected knee, because more global disease can lead to higher rates of persistent pain and conversion to total knee arthroplasty (TKA). Surgeons must exhaust all historical questions and physical examination testing to be assured that the patient's symptoms are isolated to a single compartment. In general, accepted contraindications to UKA include:

- Inflammatory arthritis
- Large fixed deformities
- Tricompartmental or bicompartmental disease
- Ligamentous laxity
- Anterior cruciate ligament deficiency (recently questioned at short-term follow-up)[7]
- Prior meniscectomy in the contralateral compartment

As an alternative, the classic indications for UKA included elderly, low-demand patients (>60 years old), weighing less than 180 pounds (body mass index <35),[8] with flexion contractures less than 10°, a good range of motion (>90°), and small overall deformities (varus deformity less than 10° or valgus deformity of less than 15°).[9] Regarding surgical technique, it is prudent to choose a surgical approach that avoids IM guides in the presence of hardware in the proximal femur and/or tibia. A second consideration is in the setting of bilateral UKAs, for which instrumenting the medullary canals on both sides may not be advisable for fear of an embolic phenomenon, making EM and spacer block techniques favored in such cases. In general, the operative technique is based on the individual surgeon's preference and experience.

SURGICAL TECHNIQUE

For the described surgical techniques it is possible to perform these procedures with minimally invasive or traditional exposures, based on the surgeon's preference. In addition, a medial parapatellar, midvastus, or subvastus arthrotomy can be used to perform UKA with equal levels of success. Adequate exposure is required to ensure that surrounding soft tissue structures are appropriately protected during the procedure and that the correct final limb alignment is achieved. Both of the described techniques avoid cannulating the medullary canal and the potential associated morbidity, including additional pain, marrow emboli cartilage damage, and postoperative bleeding from the canal.

Spacer Block Technique

When using spacer blocks to achieve flexion and extension balance and guide the bony resections, the tibia cut must be the first step of the surgical technique. An EM tibial cutting guide (as in a TKA) is placed along the lower limb and set to achieve a neutral or slightly undercorrected cut with a posterior slope of 5° to 7° (**Fig. 1**). The cutting guide lies proximally just medial to the tibial tubercle, and distally it follows the tibial crest to be positioned in the middle of the plafond (parallel to the mechanical axis of the tibia). In the sagittal plane, depending on the tibial guide used, the jig is parallel or adjusted to achieve the appropriate tibial slope. In cases with an initial 5° to 10° flexion contracture, it is suggested to make the proximal tibial resection with less posterior slope to preferentially open the extension gap greater than the flexion gap.

With the guide in place, the horizontal limb of the tibia is cut using a sagittal saw, with a typical depth of resection set at approximately 4 mm, based on the supplied stylus (see **Fig. 1**). The vertical limb is then made by paralleling the lateral aspect of the medial femoral condyle or the medial aspect of the lateral femoral condyle, for a medial or lateral UKA, respectively. It is important to adequately lateralize or medialize the vertical cut close to the tibial spine to provide enough support for the tibial tray and to avoid undersizing this implant. A notch osteophyte sometimes needs to be removed to ensure that the blade of the reciprocating saw is parallel to the femoral condyle and as close to the tibial spine as possible. Alignment guides are available to check the cut and a caliper can be used to measure the thickness of the tibial bone that is removed. The medial or lateral meniscus is then excised with gentle traction placed on the leg with the knee in extension.

A spacer block of the appropriate size is then placed and the knee is repositioned into full extension (**Fig. 2**). The goal is to ensure that the flexion and extension gaps are balanced with a spacer block of the same thickness. Limb alignment can be assessed with the attachment of targeting guides and alignment rods to ensure that the desired mechanical axis is obtained (**Fig. 3**). The distal femoral cutting guide is attached to the spacer block and pinned in place (**Fig. 4**). The distal femoral resection is then started with the knee in extension and completed in flexion as the spacer block is removed.

Balance of the flexion and extension gaps is then evaluated using spacer blocks and the tibia and femur are sized using the appropriate sizing guides (**Fig. 5**). The femoral finishing guide is placed with the paddles under the posterior femoral condyle and the anterior aspect set to have 2 to 3 mm of bone showing below the cartilage tidemark point (**Fig. 6**). The anterior portion of the guide should be up to, but not overhanging, the femoral condyle and posteriorly the guide should come to the edge of the femoral condyle at the notch. This positioning ensures that the femoral component parallels the tibial surface. As an alternative, the smallest spacer block (~8 mm) can be placed under the femoral finishing guide to set the cutting block parallel to the underlying tibial

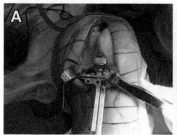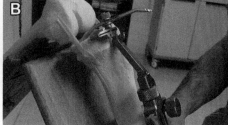

Fig. 1. (*A*) The EM tibial guide placed to over the leg and set for a resection perpendicular to the mechanical axis of the tibia with approximately 5° to 7° of posterior slope dialed into the jig. (*B*) Saw bones showing the proximal tibial resection level being set at 4 mm on the medial side for a varus knee.

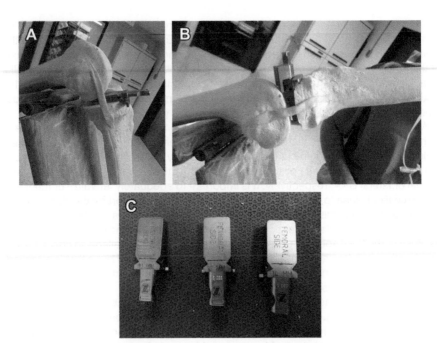

Fig. 2. Appropriate-sized spacer block is placed in flexion and extension to ensure that the correct ligamentous tension is achieved in both positions (*A, B*). Several options exist for the thickness of the spacer blocks (*C*).

surface. The finishing cuts are made and lug holes drilled for the femur and the tibia. The tibial implant should be sized to fill the space of the proximal tibia without any overhang of the trial component (**Fig. 7**). All trials are placed and balance assessed in flexion and extension with components in place. Supplemental drill holes using a 3.2-mm drill bit are made into the proximal tibia and distal femur before cementing the implants in place. The final components are cemented into place and a trial polyethylene is inserted to allow the cement to harden under pressure.

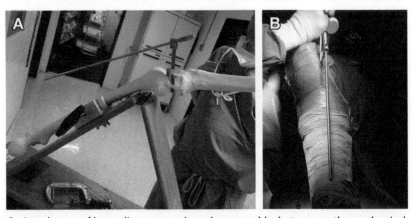

Fig. 3. Attachment of long alignment rods to the spacer blocks to assess the mechanical axis based on a marker placed at the center of the hip proximally (*A*) and the center of the plafond distally (*B*).

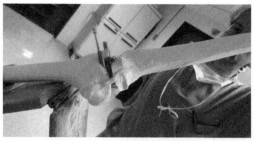

Fig. 4. The distal femoral cutting guide is placed on the tibial cut block and pinned in place in extension. The cut is initiated in extension with care taken to not plunge posteriorly with the saw blade. The remainder of the cut is completed with the knee in flexion.

True EM Technique

In the true EM technique, the distal femoral and proximal tibial cuts are linked in extension and limb alignment is set before committing to any bony cuts. Alignment is achieved first by manually correcting the limb based on soft tissue tension and surgical releases. In order to check alignment during surgery, fluoroscopy can be used before starting the surgery to place an electrocardiogram lead over the center of the femoral head. The tibial cutting guide is then placed over the leg with the EM tower attachment set for the anticipated bony resection of the distal femur (**Fig. 8**). While correcting the lower extremity to neutral with a valgus force for a medial UKA, the paddle is dialed up to meet the distal femoral condyle (this now holds the gap open). The distal femoral cutting guide is then pinned in place in full extension and the cut initiated and completed in flexion as described earlier (**Fig. 9**). The tibial resection is completed in the coronal and sagittal planes and the bony blocks are excised. The remainder of the femoral and tibial preparation occurs similar to the description for the spacer block technique.

OUTCOMES

It has long been suggested that the outcome of UKA is related to achieving the appropriate postoperative mechanical axis, with correction to neutral or slight

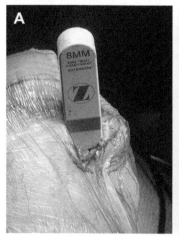
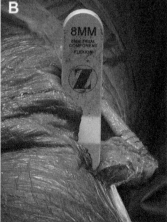

Fig. 5. Spacer blocks are placed to ensure that the flexion (*A*) and extension gaps (*B*) are symmetric.

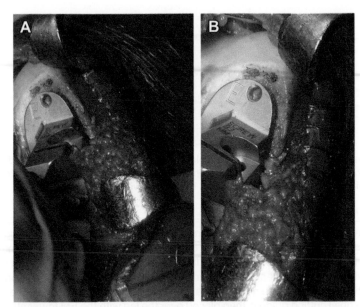

Fig. 6. The distal femur is sized and the finishing guide positioned with the paddle beneath the posterior femoral condyles (*A*) and the anterior portion of the guide lying 2 to 3 mm beneath the tidemark point of the cartilage (*B*).

undercorrection in either varus or valgus, for a medial or lateral UKA, respectively.[10] IM guides can be used in UKA, but they can be limited in their accuracy based on the rod diameter, rod length, and starting point for insertion of the guide.[11] Ma and colleagues[11] found a consistent bias toward excessive flexion and valgus with the use of an IM guide. Based on some of these inherent difficulties using IM guides, either technique described in this article can be used to circumvent such potential inaccuracies. Fisher and colleagues[12] compared EM and IM techniques for the distal femoral cuts in UKA in a retrospective manner. They found no significant differences between the two techniques; however, both were less reliable for overall alignment compared with standard TKA instrumentation.

Recent studies have reported satisfactory results with UKA using the EM techniques for bone preparation. Biswal and Brighton[13] reported on 128 UKAs using EM tibial and femoral guides with a less invasive surgical technique. They found a 92.2% survival

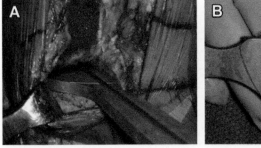
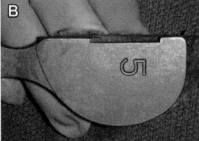

Fig. 7. The tibia is sized to ensure that maximal coverage of the plateau (*B*) is achieved without any overhang of the component into the adjacent tissues (*A*).

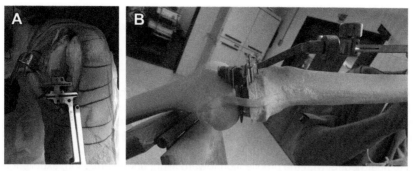

Fig. 8. The true EM tibial jig is placed over the leg (*A*) and the distal paddle is dialed out to meet the femoral condyle while the leg is being held in a neutral position by an assistant (*B*).

rate at a mean of 5.7 years' follow-up, with 92 of 98 patients reporting satisfactory results. Although modern UKA results have afforded high rates of success and patient satisfaction, outcome data must be tempered by the availability of only mid-term and short- term follow-up. Long-term follow-up is necessary to determine whether patients undergoing modern surgery will continue to have success rates rivaling those of TKA.

COMPLICATIONS

Potential complications after UKA include periprosthetic fracture, bearing dislocation, wear/osteolysis, and component fracture.[14] Tibial periprosthetic fractures have been reported in up to 4.8% of cases and can be avoided by careful and limited placement of pin holes associated with the cutting guides.[14,15] Bearing dislocations are more common with lateral UKAs and have been reported in up to 10% of cases with mobile bearing articular surfaces.[14] Additional complications have been minimized with modern component designs that are more resilient, as well as with improvements in polyethylene manufacture.

UKA revision is typically a result of failure caused by wear (12%), loosening (45%), subsidence (3.6%), arthritis progression (15%), infection (1.9%), technical problems (11.5%; eg, patella impingement and bearing dislocation), or unexplained pain

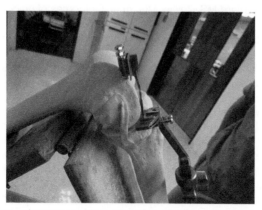

Fig. 9. The distal femoral cutting guide is pinned in place in full extension and the cut initiated and completed in flexion.

(5.5%).[16] Complications specific to the EM technique have not been described in the literature and the issues described earlier may occur in equal magnitude regardless of the technical aspects of the bony preparation.

SUMMARY

UKA surgery is a successful and reproducible procedure. The use of EM techniques to achieve component position and ligamentous balance is a safe and simple means to complete a UKA. By not having to cannulate the medullary canals, this technique promises to reduce blood loss, swelling, and malpositioning based on the IM guide insertion point. In respecting the technical principles of restoring the mechanical axis to near neutral with the predilection toward slight undercorrection, excellent outcomes can be achieved.

REFERENCES

1. Spahn G, Hofmann GO, von Engelhardt LV, et al. The impact of a high tibial valgus osteotomy and unicondylar medial arthroplasty on the treatment for knee osteoarthritis: a meta-analysis. Knee Surg Sports Traumatol Arthrosc 2011;21(1):96–112.
2. Heyse TJ, Khefacha A, Peersman G, et al. Survivorship of UKA in the middle-aged. Knee 2012;19(5):585–91.
3. Koskinen E, Paavolainen P, Eskelinen A, et al. Unicondylar knee replacement for primary osteoarthritis: a prospective follow-up study of 1,819 patients from the Finnish Arthroplasty Register. Acta Orthop 2007;78(1):128–35.
4. Svard UC, Price AJ. Oxford medial unicompartmental knee arthroplasty. A survival analysis of an independent series. J Bone Joint Surg Br 2001;83(2):191–4.
5. Geller JA, Yoon RS, Macaulay W. Unicompartmental knee arthroplasty: a controversial history and a rationale for contemporary resurgence. J Knee Surg 2008; 21(1):7–14.
6. Kim KT, Lee S, Kim TW, et al. The influence of postoperative tibiofemoral alignment on the clinical results of unicompartmental knee arthroplasty. Knee Surg Relat Res 2012;24(2):85–90.
7. Boissonneault A, Pandit H, Pegg E, et al. No difference in survivorship after unicompartmental knee arthroplasty with or without an intact anterior cruciate ligament. Knee Surg Sports Traumatol Arthrosc 2012. [Epub ahead of print].
8. Bonutti PM, Goddard MS, Zywiel MG, et al. Outcomes of unicompartmental knee arthroplasty stratified by body mass index. J Arthroplasty 2011;26(8):1149–53.
9. Kozinn SC, Scott R. Unicondylar knee arthroplasty. J Bone Joint Surg Am 1989; 71(1):145–50.
10. Psychoyios V, Crawford RW, O'Connor JJ, et al. Wear of congruent meniscal bearings in unicompartmental knee arthroplasty: a retrieval study of 16 specimens. J Bone Joint Surg Br 1998;80(6):976–82.
11. Ma B, Long W, Rudan JF, et al. Three-dimensional analysis of alignment error in using femoral intramedullary guides in unicompartmental knee arthroplasty. J Arthroplasty 2006;21(2):271–8.
12. Fisher DA, Watts M, Davis KE. Implant position in knee surgery: a comparison of minimally invasive, open unicompartmental, and total knee arthroplasty. J Arthroplasty 2003;18(7 Suppl 1):2–8.
13. Biswal S, Brighton RW. Results of unicompartmental knee arthroplasty with cemented, fixed-bearing prosthesis using minimally invasive surgery. J Arthroplasty 2010;25(5):721–7.

14. Vince KG, Cyran LT. Unicompartmental knee arthroplasty: new indications, more complications? J Arthroplasty 2004;19(4 Suppl 1):9–16.
15. Berger RA, Nedeff DD, Barden RM, et al. Unicompartmental knee arthroplasty. Clinical experience at 6- to 10-year followup. Clin Orthop Relat Res 1999;(367): 50–60.
16. Epinette JA, Brunschweiler B, Mertl P, et al. Unicompartmental knee arthroplasty modes of failure: wear is not the main reason for failure: a multicentre study of 418 failed knees. Orthop Traumatol Surg Res 2012;98(Suppl 6):S124–30.

Unicondylar Knee Arthroplasty
Intramedullary Technique

Albert S.M. Dunn, DO[a], Stephanie C. Petterson, PhD[a],
Kevin D. Plancher, MD, MS, FACS, FAAOS[a,b,c],*

KEYWORDS

- Unicondylar knee arthroplasty • Intramedullary technique • Intramedullary guide
- Partial knee replacement • Femur first technique • Unicompartmental arthritis
- Arthritis • Knee kinematics

KEY POINTS

- Use of an intramedullary femoral alignment guide for unicompartmental arthroplasty is a reliable, reproducible technique.
- Use of intramedullary alignment for partial knee replacements mimics the distal femoral preparation of total knee arthroplasty, familiar to many surgeons, improving the likelihood of successful outcomes.
- The distal femur cut provides increased working space for more accurate proximal tibial resection and also allows a flexion contracture or a non-passively correctable contracture of 15° or more to be treated successfully with a UKA in carefully selected patients.
- UKA with intramedullary instrumentation is amenable to minimally invasive surgical approaches.

INTRODUCTION

Unicondylar knee arthroplasty (UKA) has evolved substantially since its conceptual introduction by McKeever and MacIntosh in the late 1950s.[1,2] Although early results with UKA were unpredictable, this procedure restores native knee kinematics and, according to some investigators, yields patient satisfaction superior to total knee arthroplasty (TKA).[3–7] Advances in prosthetic design, bearing surface technology,[8] and surgical instrumentation have rendered excellent results in recent literature. Long-term survivorship has been reported to be as high as 98% 10 years after surgery.[9–13]

There is a general consensus that implant positioning is key to long-term survival of unicondylar arthroplasties in addition to proper patient selection.[14–16] In traditional extramedullary or spacer block techniques, the femoral cutting block is positioned

[a] Orthopaedic Foundation for Active Lifestyles, Greenwich, CT, USA; [b] Plancher Orthopaedics & Sports Medicine, 1160 Park Avenue, New York, NY 10128, USA; [c] Department of Orthopaedics, Albert Einstein College of Medicine, New York, NY, USA
* Corresponding author.
E-mail address: kplancher@plancherortho.com

Clin Sports Med 33 (2014) 87–104
http://dx.doi.org/10.1016/j.csm.2013.08.004
0278-5919/14/$ – see front matter © 2014 Elsevier Inc. All rights reserved.

freehand after the proximal tibial cut has been made. These methods have been associated with radiographic inaccuracies in prosthesis positioning in up to 30% of cases.[17] With intramedullary (IM) femoral guide instrumentation, the femoral cut is made first. Cadaveric models have confirmed that the use of IM instrumentation yields superior radiographic results in coronal alignment of the femoral component, sagittal alignment of tibial component, and overall satisfaction with prosthesis positioning.[18] We encourage use of the long IM rod for all procedures when possible. Insertion of the short IM rod in UKA per the manufacturer's guidelines may decrease the accuracy of the anatomic axis[1]; however, newer techniques and instrumentation have the ability to restore knee kinematics matching that of the native knee when the short IM rod must be used.[5,19] Furthermore, IM instrumentation for UKA mimics that of TKA, offering a more familiar operative experience for the orthopedic surgeon.[20]

PREOPERATIVE EVALUATION AND MODERN SELECTION CRITERIA

Patient selection has been a topic of debate. Criteria described by Kozinn and Scott were rigorous leaving most potential surgical candidates no other option than TKA.[21,22] Previous research has shown discrepancies in expected outcomes between patients and surgeons.[23] As a result, postoperative expectations must be discussed and managed preoperatively throughout the decision-making process to improve patient satisfaction.

Thoughts are evolving that there is no ideal candidate for UKA and an individualized approach must be taken by the surgeon. Recently expanded inclusion criteria have made this a viable option for the young, active patient seeking pain relief and return to activities without compromising the prosthesis or outcomes.[24–26] A diagnosis of osteonecrosis or osteoarthritis (OA) (**Fig. 1**)[27] in the medial or lateral compartment of the knee is understood, but weight, age, and presence or absence of the anterior cruciate ligament (ACL) must all be critically assessed.

Patients must complain of isolated knee pain to a single side of the knee with the 1-finger test (eg, ask the patient to point with 1 finger to the area of pain) (**Fig. 2**). In the case of a dual-sided loss of joint space or magnetic resonance imaging (MRI) evidence of grade IV Outerbridge OA, pain or discomfort, if present, going up stairs must match the side of pain in order to be considered a candidate for UKA. Complaints of pain going downstairs with narrowing on the medial side with grade IV Outerbridge OA yields excellent medial-sided UKA results. Patients with controlled inflammatory arthropathies are also good candidates, in our experience.

A thorough physical examination should include a full radiographic examination (eg, weight-bearing anteroposterior, lateral, posteroanterior 45° Rosenberg, and patellar views, and long leg alignment films). Radiographic inspection includes noting anteromedial joint line changes on lateral plain film radiograph for a varus knee (Ahlback stage 3 or 4) (**Fig. 3**)[28] and anterolateral joint line changes for a valgus knee (**Fig. 4**). Radiographic evidence of mild degenerative changes in the contralateral compartment can be present and still result in a successful UKA if the MRI does not reveal grade IV Outerbridge changes. Patellofemoral joint disease should be ignored regardless of Outerbridge classification if it is addressed with a patelloplasty intraoperatively.[29,30] Tibial pseudosubluxation should be a red flag to avoid failure.

Preoperative images allow visualization and measurement of angular deformities to determine the appropriate surgical plan and may even prove TKA to be the treatment of choice in some cases. Preoperative films are also used to template the prosthesis and to determine the mechanical axis for UKA to avoid overcorrecting alignment and risking failure.

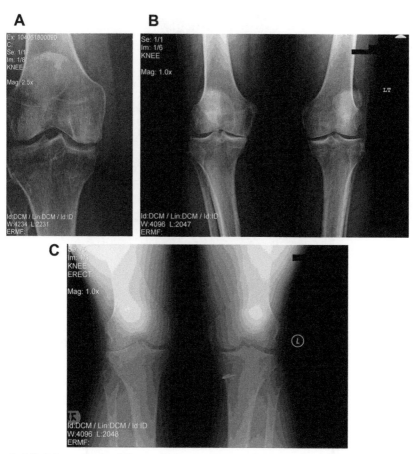

Fig. 1. (*A*) Osteonecrosis of the medial compartment. Preoperative posteroanterior notch view of avascular necrosis of the medial femoral condyle. (*B*) Medial compartment osteoarthritis. Preoperative anteroposterior view of medial compartment osteoarthritis. (*C*) Lateral compartment osteoarthritis. Preoperative posteroanterior view of lateral compartment osteoarthritis in a 58-year-old man.

A flexible, passively correctable, varus or valgus deformity of up to 15° on physical examination or stress view radiographs is acceptable, in our hands. In addition, a flexion contracture of up to 15° can be overcome in the operating room with an appropriate cut of the distal femur and tibia. A flexion range of motion (ROM) of 90°can even yield an outcome of 130° or more in many patients, with return to sport in rare circumstances.

SURGICAL TECHNIQUE

Operative setup, skin preparation, and draping for UKA using an IM technique are similar to TKA. We require all patients to wash their whole body with Hibiclens or Phisohex 1 week before surgery. The Zimmer Unicompartmental High-Flex Knee System (ZUK; Zimmer, Warsaw, IN) has yielded excellent results in the Australian registry, outperforming its predecessor, the M/G (M/G; Zimmer, Warsaw, IN) at 1, 3, and 5 years in terms of revision rates.[31] Many other accomplished surgeons have reported excellent midterm and some long-term results with this prosthesis.

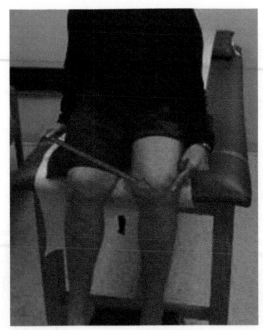

Fig. 2. The 1-finger test. On physical examination, the patient identifies the area of pain with 1 finger.

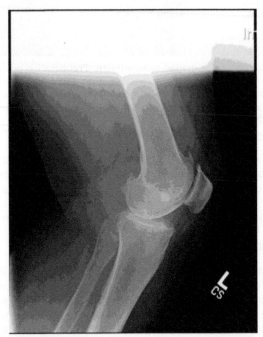

Fig. 3. Lateral plain radiographs of a varus knee requiring medial unicompartmental knee arthroplasty.

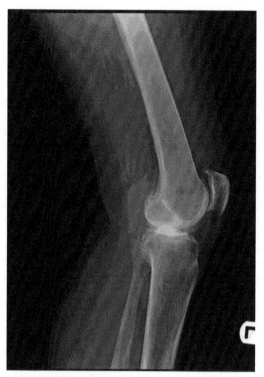

Fig. 4. Lateral plain radiographs of a valgus knee showing anterolateral joint line changes.

SURGICAL APPROACH

Minimally invasive surgical techniques are really a misnomer but have gained popularity with the general public. The size of implants restricts the ability to place the prosthesis with arthroscopic assistance. With the knee flexed to 45°, the skin incision, 9 cm long, should be made approximately 1.5 to 2 cm (approximately 1 fingerbreadth) medial to the superior pole of the patella, extending to the tibial crest (**Fig. 5**), for a medial UKA. For a lateral UKA, the incision is biased laterally, 8 to 10 cm over the lateral compartment. The patient's size should dictate the length of the incision to

A   B

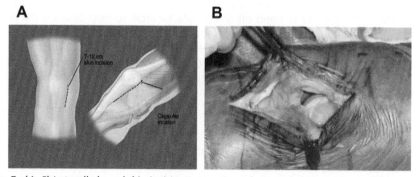

Fig. 5. (*A, B*) Laterally based skin incision approximately 9 cm, being cautious of thin tissue.

ensure accurate alignment of the prosthesis. The skin incision can be lengthened as needed for visualization if the superior aspect has a U shape, implying undue tension to the wound. The tension is relaxed at the superior or inferior apex of the incision to ensure good blood flow to the skin. Electrocautery should also be used as needed for hemostasis throughout the procedure. Hooded helmets with laminar flow can be helpful to ensure that the whole surgical team can attempt to limit any infections as well as protecting from blood being splashed inadvertently on the members of the surgical team. Dissection should occur in a single plane from the skin through subcutaneous fat and deep to Scarpa's fascia before creating a medial tissue flap. This step preserves blood supply to surrounding soft tissues and decreases the risk of postoperative wound complications.[32]

Surgical approach does not seem to alter outcomes and should be dictated by surgeon preference.[33,34] A quad-sparing parapatellar approach, a subvastus approach, or a midvastus approach can all be used for arthrotomy in a medial UKA, and a lateral parapatellar arthrotomy is used to enter the joint for a lateral UKA. We have found that by not violating the quadriceps tendon, our patients are out of bed the same day, with comfortable flexion in a continuous passive motion (CPM) device to 60°.

For a quad-sparing, midvastus approach, the arthrotomy should begin at the superior pole of the patella, dissecting in a single, full-thickness plane, and should extend proximally through the vastus medialis obliquus (VMO) or vastus lateralis obliquus (VLO) and repaired at the end of the case with an absorbable suture. We have not had any postoperative complications with denervation of the VMO or VLO and have therefore found no need for the subvastus approach.[35] Distally, the incision moves along the medial border of the patellar tendon, leaving a cuff of tissue, and over the tibial plateau, bisecting the medial or lateral meniscus in half, with the knee flexed to 45°. The knee is placed in extension when releasing the tibial tissue. From the capsular incision over the tibial plateau, the medial distal capsule is elevated subperiosteally in a single flap off of the medial aspect of the tibial plateau with a knife or key elevator in a full-thickness fashion to avoid stripping the medial collateral ligament (MCL) completely off of the bone. The distal capsular attachment to the tibial metaphysis should be maintained. Staying on bone, the dissection should be carried medially to the fibers of the deep MCL with a small cobb or key elevator, as stated earlier. The fibers of the deep MCL are elevated off the proximal tibia, taking care to maintain the distal attachment. This procedure facilitates a Z retractor placed deep to the MCL to protect the superficial MCL and all vital structures during the operation.

When exposing the lateral side of the knee with a lateral midvastus incision, it is important to note this tissue is thin, unlike the medial side of the knee. The incision as described earlier is through the VLO, moving distally through the midsection bisecting the lateral meniscus and continuing to Gerdy's tubercle. We have found that it is important to release the IT band off of Gerdy's tubercle to help balance the knee when placing a lateral UKA. The same precautions for the neurovascular structures are carried out whether on the lateral or medial side of the knee. Unlike the medial side of the knee, where flexion and external rotation help the surgeon for visualization, the figure-of-four position is helpful for the surgeon when needing extra visualization for a lateral UKA.

FAT PAD AND OSTEOPHYTE EXCISION

When beginning the operation, the synovial fluid should be examined to ensure that it is yellow and clear, with no signs of infection. The knee should be thoroughly inspected using a systematic approach. Hoffa's fat pad is a potential source of postoperative anterior knee pain, and therefore, a generous fat pad excision is recommended in the figure-of-four position for a medial UKA to decrease the risk of fat pad impingement postoperatively.[36,37] Successful excision of Hoffa's fat pad allows for improved visualization of the patellofemoral and lateral joints. Care should always be taken not to violate the patellar tendon.

Osteophyte removal from the patella is routinely performed during patellar resurfacing, similar to TKA.[38] Osteophytes are circumferentially (360°) removed with a small hand rongeur. A small rongeur and nasal rasp are then used to ensure a smooth edge. No osteophytes are removed from the femur or the tibia unless full extension is blocked or a cutting jig does not sit flush on the patient's anatomy. Removal of osteophytes from the intercondylar notch is critical to avoid ACL impingement; however, this step is not completed until the end of the procedure, along with any overhanging osteophytes on the tibia or femur, to avoid a stress riser to either bone.[39]

BONE CUTS

Bone cuts are initiated with the distal femoral cut first, followed by the proximal tibial cut, and then, the femoral posterior and chamfer cuts, with a gap-balancing technique, similar to TKA.[40] The advantages of this approach include (1) better access to the deepest portion of the tibial plateau, which is often more posterior than the tibial stylus can reach with the distal femur intact, (2) easier removal of the tibial cut bone fragment,[41] and (3) the creation of a pilot hole, in which a self-retaining patellar retractor may be placed to improve visualization.

Distal Femoral Cut Using an IM Guide

When making the distal femoral cut with the IM guide, the knee is flexed to approximately 30° and held at the ankle (**Fig. 6**). The patella is laterally translated to expose the intercondylar notch, trochlear groove, and femoral insertion of the posterior cruciate ligament (PCL). A pilot hole is drilled approximately 1 cm superior to the femoral insertion of the PCL, 1 cm medial or lateral to the apex of the intercondylar notch, and in line with the central axis of the femoral shaft.[42] If overgrowth has occurred, a rongeur is used for a better starting position. We always err with a starting hole on the side that has the disease. To avoid slipping off from the appropriate starting position, the catheter tip of the pilot drill is axially loaded through the articular cartilage until it is engaged in the subchondral bone before the drill is started. Suction is then placed

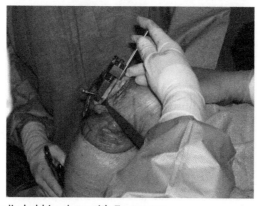

Fig. 6. Distal femur jig held in place with Z retractor.

into the drill hole to decrease IM pressures before inserting the IM guide rod.[43] The long IM rod guide with appropriate distal femoral cutting block is then inserted slowly. A short IM guide is available when a long-stem hip prosthesis is used, which is one of the reasons that we obtain 3 standing films preoperatively. A short guide is rarely used unless a bowing deformity of the femur necessitates its use.

The angulation of the cutting block should be adjusted according to preoperative templating, approximately 6° for a varus knee and 3° or 4° for a valgus knee. The cutting block should be flush with the distal femoral condyle, which is accomplished by soft tissue dissection. The posterior aspect of the cutting block is pinned in place with a long-headed, 48-mm pin, and the distal femoral cut is made down to the level of the posterior slotted pin. After the slotted pin is removed, the cut is completed (**Fig. 7**). The IM guide is removed in order to inspect the distal femoral cut. It is critical that the distal femoral cut is flat because the posterior and chamfer femoral cuts are dependent on this first cut. A large bone file from a TKA set is used. A self-retaining IM patellar retractor is placed into the IM pilot hole with the knee flexed to 90°. Alignment is exclusively obtained with this jig, and therefore, the importance of this step cannot be overemphasized. The posterior surface of the femoral jig must be perpendicular to the femur, ignoring the tibial surface. It is crucial to release the tibial surface for a medial UKA, to avoid a varus knee and a failed UKA. For a valgus knee, we advise a release of the IT band in all patients because the valgus knee heals back to bone within several weeks.

Proximal Tibial Cut with Extramedullary Guide

The extramedullary tibial guide is positioned in line with the long axis of the tibia using ankle clamps, similar to the same step in a TKA. Minimizing padding at the ankle allows for easier palpation of the distal tibia. The guide should be either medial or lateral to the tibial crest to ensure correct alignment depending on a varus or valgus knee. A lateral patellar incision is used for our valgus knees. The posterior slope should mirror the patient's native anatomy, as determined during preoperative planning. A posterior slope of approximately 5° to 7° is recommended, with a slope at a lesser degree for an ACL-deficient knee. In the presence of an extension lag, the cut should be more

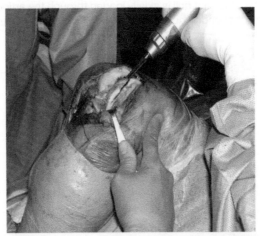

Fig. 7. Completion of distal femoral cut. It is important to protect the soft tissues when completing the distal femoral cut.

anterior than posterior, despite fears of creating hyperextension. This strategy allows the contracted hamstrings a chance to be stretched out during the early postoperative period. When proceeding in this fashion, loss of extension, common in patients 70 years or older, is not a contraindication for a UKA, in our experience (**Fig. 8**).

The cutting block is centered over the medial or lateral tibial surface without overlapping the patellar tendon to avoid cutting it with the saw. A 4-mm slotted stylus is used to measure the appropriate amount of resection on the deepest portion of the tibial plateau, which is easily visible after the resection of the distal femur has been completed. The proximal tibial cutting block should be secured with 2 headless, threaded, long pins and the extramedullary guide left in place for added security with a long-headed, threaded pin. Three pins are used to secure the tibial cutting block; there have been no postoperative stress fractures.[44]

The proximal tibial cut is made with the tibial cutting block and extramedullary guide with the knee positioned in 90°. Hyperflexion should always be avoided when completing this cut. Care is taken to protect the MCL with a Z retractor placed meticulously for a medial UKA and on the lateral side to protect vital structures for a lateral UKA. A sagittal saw with a triangular tip is used to avoid a small bone bridge on the anterolateral or medial aspect of the tibial plateau where the sagittal and proximal tibial cuts meet. The saw blade should be placed lateral or medial to the guide, hugging the medial or lateral aspect of the intercondylar notch. Extreme caution must be used when using this saw to avoid penetrating the posterior capsule. In addition, care must be taken to avoid undercutting the tibial spine when vertically pushing to avoid a fracture.

When the cut of bone is removed as 1 piece, it can be used as a guide to determine the proper tibial tray size. To successfully do this, a cobb is placed on top with a 1.27-cm (0.5-inch) flat osteotome underneath. It is essential not to wedge the osteotome. The leg should be placed in external rotation and 90° flexion and the cobb used on the medial side to remove the bone fragment. For a lateral UKA, a figure-of-four position can be used to successfully complete this step. When the fragment is difficult to remove, a knife can be used to remove the capsular meniscal attachments, which should have been removed at the beginning of the procedure.

It is important to verify the gaps at this point in the procedure in order to decrease the odds of a gap imbalance when trialing components. An 8-mm or 10-mm spacer guide is placed to ensure that full extension has been maintained as well as no flexion tightness.

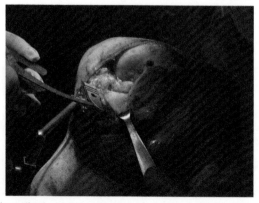

Fig. 8. Extramedullary tibial guided positioned for a medial UKA. The angel wing verifies the level of cut with soft tissue protection.

Posterior Femoral and Chamfer Cuts

The final cuts are made with the knee flexed to 90°. The appropriate-sized femoral sizer/finishing guide is selected. When determining the appropriate size, 2 mm of cut bone should be exposed anteriorly from the previously made distal femoral cut. The posterior boot of the guide should contact the cartilage of the posterior femoral condyle. Oversizing this component leads to patellar impingement.[45] Once the guide is flush with the previously made distal femoral cut, the femoral finishing guide is pinned in place anteriorly (**Fig. 9**). It is important to line this jig up with the flat cut surface of the tibia to avoid edge loading. The jig is rotated to the posterior aspect of the finishing guide until it is collinear with the proximal tibial cut and headed, threaded long pins are placed to secure the cutting block. Both peg holes are now drilled to a positive stop on the drill. The chamfer and posterior femoral cuts should be made sequentially through the guide. The chamfer cut must be exact and often requires removal of 1 pin and placing it in a different hole. We recommend cutting the posterior femoral cuts before the chamfer cut. The appropriate femoral trial component is placed on the prepared femoral condyle (**Fig. 10**). A headed gold pin locks the jig in place and the posterior pins are also placed. We have found that in order to avoid edge loading, we bias the femoral sizer toward the notch. With all cuts complete, a smooth, laminar spreader is placed and 1.27-cm (0.5-inch) curved osteotome is used to remove all posterior osteophytes to gain high flexion. Any remaining meniscus is excised and the posterior joint is inspected for any loose bodies.

TRIALING COMPONENTS AND BALANCING GAPS

The key to a successful UKA is a well-aligned prosthesis, restoring the mechanical axis to neutral (or slight undercorrection), and having appropriate ligamentous tension in both flexion and extension without overstuffing the prosthesis. Overloading the contralateral compartment can accelerate degenerative changes.[46] The use of the spacer guide minimizes this risk by ensuring laxity in the operative compartment, as discussed earlier.

The fit of the tibial trials is best evaluated with the knee in 90° of flexion and slight external rotation. The use of the largest tibial tray possible without overhang, matching the implant size to the peripheral cortical bone, provides the most support for the implant (**Fig. 11**). Occasionally, the sagittal cut may need to be repeated, moving toward the notch to accommodate the larger tibial tray. Once the trial tibial tray is inserted, rotational alignment is confirmed when the insertion handle is 90° to the coronal axis of the proximal tibia and no overhang is noted.

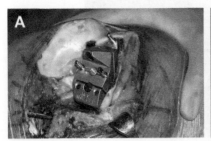
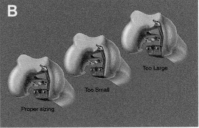

Fig. 9. (*A*) Femoral cutting block in place. It is important to appropriately size the femoral cutting block so there is no overhang. (*B*) Proper sizing of the femoral jig.

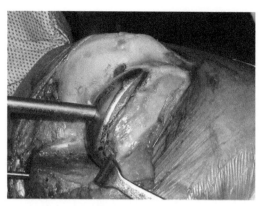

Fig. 10. Femoral trial sizing is completed before the trial component is placed on the prepared femoral surface.

A curved device is included in the set to feel around the back of the knee with the sizing guide to ensure that the correct tibial prosthesis is selected. The tibial keel is prepared with the provided keel punch and then inserted (**Fig. 12A**). It is important when creating this trough to first set it flush with the tibial cut surface, then send it posteriorly with good coverage, before drilling the 2, 20°-angled posterior tibial holes (see **Fig. 12B**). The trial femoral component and the trial polyethylene component are then inserted and the patellar retractor is removed.

After the trial components are inserted, the flexion extension gaps and tracking are evaluated. The knee is moved through its full ROM without the tension gauge to assess tracking between the femoral and tibial components. The tension gauge is then inserted, with the knee flexed to 90°. The tension gauge should slip in and out of the joint with 2 fingers and slight resistance without movement of the tibial trial on the 2-mm side. Movement of the tibial trial is an indication that the flexion gap may be too tight. This step should also be repeated with the knee in full extension. If the tibial trial moves when in extension, the extension gap may be too tight. At this point, necessary adjustments should be made to balance the gaps and properly align the components.

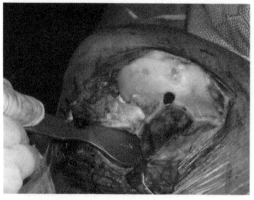

Fig. 11. Templates to find the largest tibial tray are completed.

A   **B**

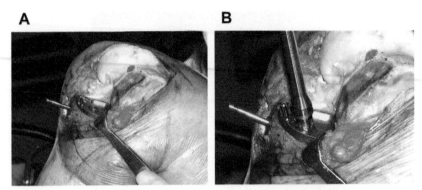

Fig. 12. (*A*) The tibial keel is placed with an appropriate tibial tray to finalize preparation of the tibial surface. (*B*) The cut tibial surface is completed, and the posterior tibial holes are prepared.

FINAL PREPARATION AND CEMENTING OF FINAL IMPLANTS

In final preparation for implant placement, the prepared bony surfaces are copiously irrigated with antibiotic solutions and the joint is reinspected for debris. The bony surfaces are dried and a 10.2-cm × 20.3-cm (4-inch × 8-inch) sponge held by a Z retractor is placed in the posterior aspect of the joint in addition to a thrombin spray. The cement should be compressed into the tibia with a finger or a ganglion knife, making sure not to place excessive cement posteriorly. Excess cement is difficult to remove after the implants are in place. We advise placing a small amount of cement only on the posterior aspect of the prosthesis and the anterior section of the tibia. The final tibial component is then inserted and impacted into place. A small, curved curette and a knife are used to remove excess cement from the posterior aspect of the joint. The process is then repeated with the femoral component, and the trial polyethylene component is placed (**Fig. 13**).

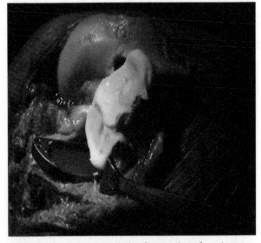

Fig. 13. The tibia is cemented in place, and the femoral surface is prepared with cement to accept the real prosthesis.

The leg is moved into extension to compress the components while the cement cures. The cement is monitored, and when appropriate, the previously packed sponge in the posterior aspect of joint is removed. Excess posterior cement should be brought into view for removal (**Fig. 14**). If the Z retractor is placed back in the joint, it should always be checked first to make sure that it does not have any excess cement. The trial polyethylene component is removed when the cement hardens, and the real polyethylene is inserted after checking the gaps (**Fig. 15**). We advise avoiding making the knee too tight. The MCL is checked in extension and flexion to ensure appropriate laxity. The wound should be copiously irrigated before closure of the incision in the surgeon's preferred standard fashion; our preference is a subcuticular monocryl (**Fig. 16**).

COMPLICATIONS AND OUTCOMES

Please see "Outcomes and Complications of Unicondylar Arthroplasty" by Della Valle et al, elsewhere in this issue for detailed outcomes and complications.

Long-term outcomes of UKA performed with IM instrumentation are good. Berger and colleagues reported 98% survivorship at 10 years and 95.7% at 13 years when conversion to TKA was used as the end point in 62 consecutive patients. When aspetic loosening was used as an end point, survivorship increased to 100% at 13 years; 80% of patients reported excellent satisfaction, 12% reported good satisfaction, and 8% reported fair satisfaction. The 2 failures were because of progression of symptomatic arthritis in other compartments, albeit at a slow progression rate of 7 and 11 years.

Patients with UKA outperform their peers with TKA on reported symptoms, activities of daily living, and sport and recreation.[47,48] Patients with UKA show greater knee ROM and report less difficulty with activities that involve bending their knee.[48,49] Body mass index (BMI, calculated as weight in kilograms divided by the square of height in meters) does not adversely affect outcomes[50] and persons with BMI greater than 35 continue to show functional improvement for at least 2 years after surgery.[51]

In a recent review of our series, 52 of 56 patients (93%) who participated in sports preoperatively and underwent UKA returned to sports within 6 months after UKA. The 3 patients who did not resume sports postoperatively did not resume sports for reasons unrelated to their knee. All patients who participated in tennis (N = 14) and skiing (N = 23) preoperatively resumed after UKA without complication.

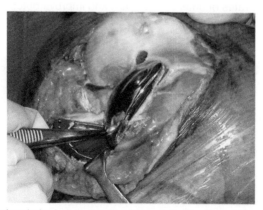

Fig. 14. The femoral and tibial components are cemented in place and any excessive cement outside the components or under the engaging locking mechanism is safely removed.

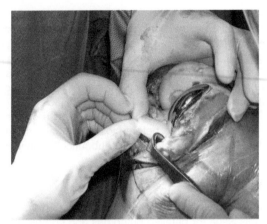

Fig. 15. The real polyethylene insert is snapped into place with an audible sound.

POSTOPERATIVE PROTOCOL AND REHABILITATION

ROM exercises are initiated immediately postoperatively in the postanesthesia care unit, and a multimodal pain control regimen is routinely used, including nonsteroidal antiinflammatory drugs and 1-time intravenous steroid intraoperatively to control swelling.[52] A Hemovac drain is also used and sewn in the knee. We have found that the number 1 complication in our patients is too much activity too fast too soon with hematoma collection. For this reason, a drain is left in for several days, and we have had no infections. A CPM device and extensive icing are used to return our patients to activities in an accelerated fashion. The drain is taken out in the office and ambulation is partial weight bearing with crutches or a walker for the octogenarians. Deep vein thrombosis prophylaxis is based on risk stratification in accordance with the recommendations from the American Academy of Orthopaedic Surgeons.[53] We prefer Coumadin for 6 weeks with thigh-high compression stockings.

A formal outpatient rehabilitation program is prescribed including wall slides and stationary bike riding without tension and the seat placed high to avoid excessive flexion starting on day 1. Emphasis is placed on ROM, restoration of normal mechanics, and strengthening of the core, hip, and quadriceps, which has been shown to decrease rates of anterior knee pain and improve outcomes.[54–56] Strength

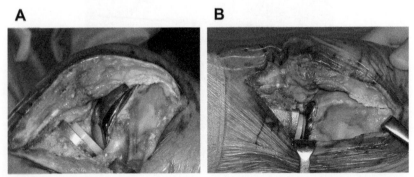

Fig. 16. Final UKA with real polyethylene liner. (*A*) Knee in full flexion. (*B*) Knee in full extension.

training is not initiated until 6 weeks postoperatively. Patients are permitted to return to their desired activities without restrictions after the completion of their physical therapy program. We allow patients to return to golf (riding in a cart) at 8 to 12 weeks, depending on swelling. Singles tennis and downhill skiing are permitted at 6 months.

SUMMARY

UKA is a reliable method of alleviating pain and restoring function in patients with knee arthritis with the appropriate indications and meticulous surgical technique. Use of IM instrumentation on the femur provides a similar operative experience to TKA, allowing most surgeons the comfort of a procedure known well to them. Preoperative goal setting and postoperative rehabilitation involving core, hip, and quadriceps strengthening are nonsurgical adjuncts, which enhance outcomes and patient satisfaction in this already successful procedure.

REFERENCES

1. McKeever DC. Tibial plateau prosthesis. Clin Orthop Relat Res 1960;18:86–95.
2. MacIntosh DL, Hunter GA. The use of the hemiarthroplasty prosthesis for advanced osteoarthritis and rheumatoid arthritis of the knee. J Bone Joint Surg Br 1972;54(2):244–55.
3. Laurencin CT, Zelicof SB, Scott RD, et al. Unicompartmental versus total knee arthroplasty in the same patient. A comparative study. Clin Orthop Relat Res 1991;(273):151–6.
4. Knutson K, Lindstrand A, Lidgren L. Survival of knee arthroplasties. A nationwide multicentre investigation of 8000 cases. J Bone Joint Surg Br 1986; 68(5):795–803.
5. Patil S, Colwell CW Jr, Ezzet KA, et al. Can normal knee kinematics be restored with unicompartmental knee replacement? J Bone Joint Surg Am 2005;87(2): 332–8.
6. Noticewala MS, Geller JA, Lee JH, et al. Unicompartmental knee arthroplasty relieves pain and improves function more than total knee arthroplasty. J Arthroplasty 2012;27(Suppl 8):99–105.
7. Rougraff BT, Heck DA, Gibson AE. A comparison of tricompartmental and unicompartmental arthroplasty for the treatment of gonarthrosis. Clin Orthop Relat Res 1991;(273):157–64.
8. Oral E, Neils AL, Rowell SL, et al. Increasing irradiation temperature maximizes vitamin E grafting and wear resistance of ultrahigh molecular weight polyethylene. J Biomed Mater Res B Appl Biomater 2013;101(3):436–40.
9. Price AJ, Waite JC, Svard U. Long-term clinical results of the medial Oxford unicompartmental knee arthroplasty. Clin Orthop Relat Res 2005;(435): 171–80.
10. Naudie D, Guerin J, Parker DA, et al. Medial unicompartmental knee arthroplasty with the Miller-Galante prosthesis. J Bone Joint Surg Am 2004;86-A(9): 1931–5.
11. Berger RA, Meneghini RM, Jacobs JJ, et al. Results of unicompartmental knee arthroplasty at a minimum of ten years of follow-up. J Bone Joint Surg Am 2005; 87(5):999–1006.
12. Argenson JN, Chevrol-Benkeddache Y, Aubaniac JM. Modern unicompartmental knee arthroplasty with cement: A three to ten-year follow-up study. J Bone Joint Surg Am 2002;84-A(12):2235–9.

13. Keblish PA, Briard JL. Mobile-bearing unicompartmental knee arthroplasty: A 2-center study with an 11-year (mean) follow-up. J Arthroplasty 2004;19(7 Suppl 2):87–94.

14. Cartier P, Sanouiller JL, Grelsamer RP. Unicompartmental knee arthroplasty surgery. 10-year minimum follow-up period. J Arthroplasty 1996;11(7):782–8.

15. Hernigou P, Deschamps G. Prothèses unicompartimentales du genou. Rev Chir Orthop Reparatrice Appar Mot 1996;82(Suppl):23–60 [in French].

16. Lootvoet L, Burton P, Himmer O, et al. A unicompartment knee prosthesis: The effect of the positioning of the tibial plate on the functional results. Acta Orthop Belg 1997;63(2):94–101.

17. Tabor OB Jr, Tabor OB. Unicompartmental arthroplasty: A long-term follow-up study. J Arthroplasty 1998;13(4):373–9.

18. Jenny JY, Boeri C. Accuracy of implantation of a unicompartmental total knee arthroplasty with 2 different instrumentations: A case-controlled comparative study. J Arthroplasty 2002;17(8):1016–20.

19. Whiteside LA, McCarthy DS. Laboratory evaluation of alignment and kinematics in a unicompartmental knee arthroplasty inserted with intramedullary instrumentation. Clin Orthop Relat Res 1992;(274):238–47.

20. Della Valle CJ, Berger RA, Rosenberg AG. Minimally invasive unicompartmental knee arthroplasty using intramedullary femoral alignment. Oper Tech Orthop 2006;16(3):186–94.

21. Stern SH, Becker MW, Insall JN. Unicondylar knee arthroplasty. An evaluation of selection criteria. Clin Orthop Relat Res 1993;(286):143–8.

22. Kozinn SC, Scott R. Unicondylar knee arthroplasty. J Bone Joint Surg Am 1989; 71(1):145–50.

23. Greene KA, Harwin SF. Maximizing patient satisfaction and functional results after total knee arthroplasty. J Knee Surg 2011;24(1):19–24.

24. Berend KR, Lombardi AV Jr. Liberal indications for minimally invasive Oxford unicondylar arthroplasty provide rapid functional recovery and pain relief. Surg Technol Int 2007;16:193–7.

25. Pennington DW, Swienckowski JJ, Lutes WB, et al. Unicompartmental knee arthroplasty in patients sixty years of age or younger. J Bone Joint Surg Am 2003; 85-A(10):1968–73.

26. Borus T, Thornhill T. Unicompartmental knee arthroplasty. J Am Acad Orthop Surg 2008;16(1):9–18.

27. Parratte S, Argenson JN, Dumas J, et al. Unicompartmental knee arthroplasty for avascular osteonecrosis. Clin Orthop Relat Res 2007;464:37–42.

28. Ahlback S. Osteoarthrosis of the knee. A radiographic investigation. Acta Radiol Diagn (Stockh) 1968;(Suppl 277):7–72.

29. Beard DJ, Pandit H, Ostlere S, et al. Pre-operative clinical and radiological assessment of the patellofemoral joint in unicompartmental knee replacement and its influence on outcome. J Bone Joint Surg Br 2007;89(12): 1602–7.

30. Outerbridge RE. The etiology of chondromalacia patellae. J Bone Joint Surg Br 1961;43-B:752–7.

31. AOA. The Australian Orthopaedic Association national joint replacement registry. Annual report. 2012.

32. Younger AS, Duncan CP, Masri BA. Surgical exposures in revision total knee arthroplasty. J Am Acad Orthop Surg 1998;6(1):55–64.

33. Aglietti P, Baldini A, Sensi L. Quadriceps-sparing versus mini-subvastus approach in total knee arthroplasty. Clin Orthop Relat Res 2006;452:106–11.

34. Bonutti PM, Zywiel MG, Ulrich SD, et al. A comparison of subvastus and midvastus approaches in minimally invasive total knee arthroplasty. J Bone Joint Surg Am 2010;92(3):575–82.
35. Dalury DF, Snow RG, Adams MJ. Electromyographic evaluation of the midvastus approach. J Arthroplasty 2008;23(1):136–40.
36. Biedert RM, Sanchis-Alfonso V. Sources of anterior knee pain. Clin Sports Med 2002;21(3):335–47, vii.
37. Kumar D, Alvand A, Beacon JP. Impingement of infrapatellar fat pad (Hoffa's disease): results of high-portal arthroscopic resection. Arthroscopy 2007; 23(11):1180–6.e1.
38. Liu ZT, Fu PL, Wu HS, et al. Patellar reshaping versus resurfacing in total knee arthroplasty–results of a randomized prospective trial at a minimum of 7 years' follow-up. Knee 2012;19(3):198–202.
39. Hoteya K, Kato Y, Motojima S, et al. Association between intercondylar notch narrowing and bilateral anterior cruciate ligament injuries in athletes. Arch Orthop Trauma Surg 2011;131(3):371–6.
40. Dennis DA, Komistek RD, Kim RH, et al. Gap balancing versus measured resection technique for total knee arthroplasty. Clin Orthop Relat Res 2010;468(1): 102–7.
41. Shakespeare D, Waite J. The Oxford medial partial knee replacement. The rationale for a femur first technique. Knee 2012;19(6):927–32.
42. Wangroongsub Y, Cherdtaweesup S. Proper entry point for femoral intramedullary guide in total knee arthroplasty. J Med Assoc Thai 2009;92(Suppl 6): S1–5.
43. Amro RR, Nazarian DG, Norris RB, et al. Suction instrumentation decreases intramedullary pressure and pulmonary embolism during total knee arthroplasty. University of Pennsylvania Orthopaedic Journal 2001;14:55–9.
44. Brumby SA, Carrington R, Zayontz S, et al. Tibial plateau stress fracture: A complication of unicompartmental knee arthroplasty using 4 guide pinholes. J Arthroplasty 2003;18(6):809–12.
45. Hernigou P, Deschamps G. Patellar impingement following unicompartmental arthroplasty. J Bone Joint Surg Am 2002;84-A(7):1132–7.
46. Koeck FX, Beckmann J, Luring C, et al. Evaluation of implant position and knee alignment after patient-specific unicompartmental knee arthroplasty. Knee 2011;18(5):294–9.
47. Walton NP, Jahromi I, Lewis PL, et al. Patient-perceived outcomes and return to sport and work: TKA versus mini-incision unicompartmental knee arthroplasty. J Knee Surg 2006;19(2):112–6.
48. Lygre SH, Espehaug B, Havelin LI, et al. Pain and function in patients after primary unicompartmental and total knee arthroplasty. J Bone Joint Surg Am 2010; 92(18):2890–7.
49. Amin AK, Patton JT, Cook RE, et al. Unicompartmental or total knee arthroplasty?: Results from a matched study. Clin Orthop Relat Res 2006;451:101–6.
50. Naal FD, Neuerburg C, Salzmann GM, et al. Association of body mass index and clinical outcome 2 years after unicompartmental knee arthroplasty. Arch Orthop Trauma Surg 2009;129(4):463–8.
51. Thompson SA, Liabaud B, Nellans KW, et al. Factors associated with poor outcomes following unicompartmental knee arthroplasty: Redefining the "classic" indications for surgery. J Arthroplasty 2013; Mar 21. [Epub ahead of print].
52. Parvizi J, Miller AG, Gandhi K. Multimodal pain management after total joint arthroplasty. J Bone Joint Surg Am 2011;93(11):1075–84.

53. Mont MA, Jacobs JJ, Boggio LN, et al. Preventing venous thromboembolic disease in patients undergoing elective hip and knee arthroplasty. J Am Acad Orthop Surg 2011;19(12):768–76.

54. Earl JE, Hoch AZ. A proximal strengthening program improves pain, function, and biomechanics in women with patellofemoral pain syndrome. Am J Sports Med 2011;39(1):154–63.

55. Shirey M, Hurlbutt M, Johansen N, et al. The influence of core musculature engagement on hip and knee kinematics in women during a single leg squat. Int J Sports Phys Ther 2012;7(1):1–12.

56. Chiu JK, Wong YM, Yung PS, et al. The effects of quadriceps strengthening on pain, function, and patellofemoral joint contact area in persons with patellofemoral pain. Am J Phys Med Rehabil 2012;91(2):98–106.

Mobile-bearing Unicondylar Knee Arthroplasty: The Oxford Experience

Jason M. Hurst, MD*, Keith R. Berend, MD

KEYWORDS

- Knee • Mobile bearing • Unicompartmental arthroplasty • Oxford

KEY POINTS

- Partial knee arthroplasty is growing in popularity, especially in active adults and those patients seeking less invasive surgery and rapid recovery.
- The mobile-bearing, fully congruent design of the Oxford knee has less wear than fixed-bearing designs.
- The long-term outcome data of the Oxford knee rival those of total knee arthroplasty without the inherent morbidity, mortality, and other risks. This success of the Oxford has begun to challenge the dogma surrounding total knee arthroplasty.
- The Oxford partial knee is ideal for outpatient procedures.
- The modern design and instrumentation allows for minimally invasive implantation.

INTRODUCTION

The past 2 decades have seen a resurgence of interest in unicompartmental knee arthroplasty (UKA) for the treatment of isolated knee arthritis. The resurgence of medial UKA is in part due to a movement toward less invasive techniques, quicker recovery, less overall morbidity, and preservation of normal knee kinematics.[1–4] This growth in popularity, combined with recent reports of long-term success with medial UKA, has also begun to challenge the dogmatic belief that total knee arthroplasty (TKA) is the gold standard treatment of all knee arthrosis.[5–7]

The Oxford mobile-bearing UKA (Biomet, Inc, Warsaw, IN) is an implant with a unique design that has a spherical femoral component, a polished flat tibial component, and a fully congruent polyethylene meniscal bearing. This design is in sharp contrast with most medial UKA devices that use an aspherical femoral component and fixed polyethylene tibial component. The traditional fixed-bearing design creates

Funding Sources: Biomet.
Conflicts of Interest: Biomet.
Joint Implant Surgeon Inc, 7277 Smith's Mill Road, Suite 200, New Albany, OH 43054, USA
* Corresponding author.
E-mail address: JasonHurst@mac.com

Clin Sports Med 33 (2014) 105–121
http://dx.doi.org/10.1016/j.csm.2013.06.004

the opportunity for polyethylene wear secondary to high-contact stresses over low surface area.[8] The fully congruent mobile-bearing design of the Oxford UKA has been shown to reduce polyethylene wear to 0.01 to 0.02 mm per year while maintaining more normal knee kinematics.[9]

OXFORD DESIGN HISTORY AND RATIONALE

Goodfellow and colleagues[10] developed the concept of the Oxford knee in the early 1970s. The initial premise of the design was to reduce polyethylene wear by reproducing the congruent nature of the native meniscus. This congruent design increased the contact area but greatly reduced the contact stresses. However, in order to achieve full congruency on both interfaces with a solid polyethylene meniscus, the femoral side needed to be spherical and the tibial side needed to be flat.

The implant was originally used as a bicompartmental knee replacement with poor survivorship.[11] The survivorship of the Oxford knee was markedly improved once its use was limited to the medial compartment of ligamentously stable knees with bone-on-bone osteoarthritis.[5] White and colleagues[12] defined this distinct pattern of medial disease as anteromedial osteoarthritis and only observed this pattern in patients with an intact anterior cruciate ligament (ACL). Those patients with ACL deficiency tended to have a posteromedial wear patterns secondary to the chronic anterior subluxation of the medial tibia that occurs when the ACL is incompetent. This pattern of anteromedial osteoarthritis is now the primary indication for a medial Oxford UKA.

The Oxford UKA has undergone a series of modifications since the 1970s. However, the original concepts remain unchanged since its initial development (**Fig. 1**A). Femoral milling was developed in 1987 to accurately and safely prepare the medial femoral condyle and allow for minimally invasive implantation (see **Fig. 1**B). The third phase of development in the late 1990s created additional femoral component sizes and a more anatomic meniscal bearing that improved tracking and diminished bearing impingement and rotation (see **Fig. 1**C). This phase III design also incorporated anatomic femoral sizes and a novel instrumentation platform specifically designed for minimally invasive implantation.

The most recent phase of Oxford development started in 2009 and focused on improving the reliability of the instrumentation, eliminating impingement of the meniscal bearing, and slight modifications to the femoral design (see **Fig. 1**D). The new Microplasty Instrumentation (Biomet, Inc, Warsaw, IN) of the Oxford UKA uses an intramedullary reference for preparing the femur and a reproducible stylus to create a more consistent tibial resection. The new twin-peg femoral design maintains the same spherical design concept but has an additional peg for rotational stability; a longer radius of curvature to maintain bearing congruency in high flexion angles; and smoother, rounded edges to reduce soft tissue irritation and impingement (see **Fig. 1**D).

INDICATIONS

The typical radiographic evaluation of an Oxford UKA candidate is seen in **Fig. 2**. It is important to notice that, in this case example, the knee corrects to a normal valgus alignment with valgus stress and that the lateral joint space is maintained. **Fig. 3** shows patients who are not candidates for UKA based on the failure of the valgus stress film and the presence of a posteromedial wear pattern in ACL deficiency.

The indications for medial Oxford UKA as defined by Goodfellow and colleagues[10] are:

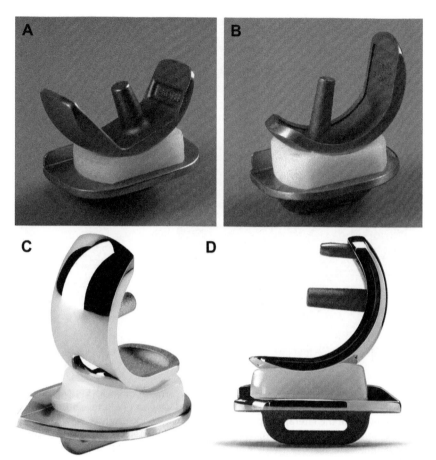

Fig. 1. The Oxford has undergone 4 series of development: (A) phase 1 (1970s), (B) phase 2 (1980s), (C) phase 3 (1990s), (D) twin peg microplasty (2009). (*Courtesy of* Biomet, Inc., Warsaw IN; with permission.)

- Bone-on-bone anteromedial osteoarthritic wear pattern
- Ligamentously normal knee with an intact ACL
- Correctable varus deformity
- Well-maintained, normal lateral joint space on valgus stress view radiograph (see **Fig. 2E; Fig. 4**)

The traditional Kozinn and colleagues[13] inclusion criteria are not considered the current indications for the Oxford UKA.[14] Contrary to popular dogma, mild to moderate patellofemoral disease is not considered a contraindication unless there is severe lateral patellar facet wear and grooving of the lateral trochlear ridge.[5,15] There has been no study that links mild to moderate patellofemoral disease to failure of UKA or a predominating reason for conversion to TKA. There are multiple reports that support ignoring the patellofemoral disease in the presence of anteromedial osteoarthritis of the tibiofemoral joint.[5–7,16,17]

Although all surgeons agree that knee replacement surgery is reserved for elderly patients with end-stage osteoarthritis who have failed conservative measures, there is currently no limitation with respect to patient age as long as the patient has

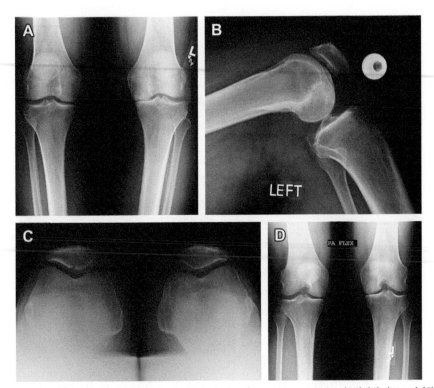

Fig. 2. The typical radiographic work-up includes the anteroposterior (AP) (*A*), lateral (*B*), and sunrise views (*C*). The posteroanterior (PA) flexed view can help reveal bone-on-bone disease and evaluate the lateral compartment (*D*). However, the essential view is the valgus stress view, which thoroughly determines the integrity of the lateral compartment cartilage (*E*). Postoperative images (*F, G*) show a stable implant with appropriate correction of the alignment.

bone-on-bone anteromedial disease and meets the inclusion criteria.[18] Obesity was once seen as a contraindication to UKA; however, with the metal-backed design of the Oxford, obesity is not considered a contraindication.[19,20]

The current list of contraindicated conditions includes[10]:

- Inflammatory arthropathy
- Previous high tibial osteotomy (opening or closing wedge)
- ACL deficiency
- Medial collateral ligament (MCL) contracture with inability to correct the varus deformity
- Weight-bearing cartilage wear of the lateral compartment
- Severe patellofemoral arthrosis with lateral facet disease, lateral subluxation, and trochlear grooving

Other conditions that can be successfully treated with Oxford UKA include avascular necrosis (AVN) of the medial femoral condyle, posttraumatic medial compartment arthritis, and chronic medial femoral condyle osteochondritis dissecans (OCD) (**Fig. 5**).[21] In order to ensure adequate femoral component fixation, careful attention must be paid to the femoral bone stock in cases of AVN and large OCD lesions. In

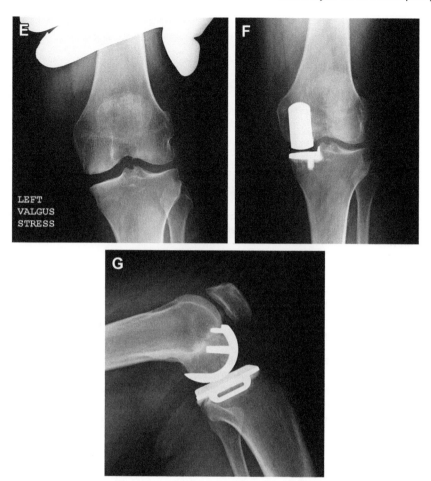

Fig. 2. (*continued*)

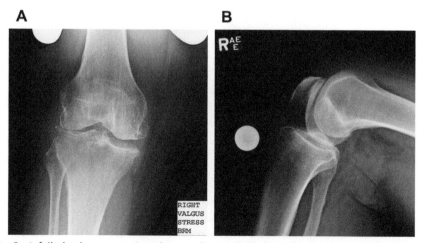

Fig. 3. A failed valgus stress view shows collapse of the lateral compartment (*A*). A posteromedial wear pattern seen on the lateral view can indicate chronic ACL insufficiency (*B*).

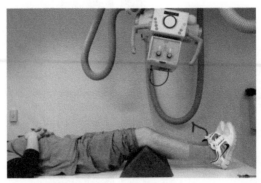

Fig. 4. The valgus stress radiograph is performed by aiming the x-ray beam with 10° of tilt at the joint line of the knee flexed to 20° over a bolster. Light valgus pressure is applied using lead gloves.

the rare cases of medial compartment traumatic arthritis, the knee must still be ligamentously stable and the deformity correctable without MCL contracture.

SURGICAL TECHNIQUE

Most Oxford UKAs can be performed as an outpatient procedure if the patient meets medical criteria and the anesthesia is adequate. The typical anesthesia is general anesthesia coupled with a peripheral nerve block, short-acting spinal injection, and/ or local pericapsular injection. The patient is typically positioned in a hanging leg holder that flexes the hip to approximately 30° and allows the operative knee to flex to 135° (**Fig. 6**).

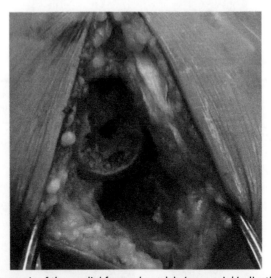

Fig. 5. Avascular necrosis of the medial femoral condyle is a special indication for the Oxford but care must be taken to remove all necrotic bone and allow the defect to be filled with a significant amount of cement.

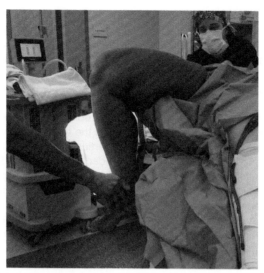

Fig. 6. The typical Oxford setup includes a hanging leg holder that flexes the hip approximately 30° and still allows the knee to be flexed to 135°.

A paramedial incision is made from the superomedial edge of the patella to the medial border of the tibial tubercle (**Fig. 7**). This incision can be extended proximally and distally in cases of intraoperative conversion to TKA. The anteromedial portion of the tibia needs to be exposed for tibial resection; however, the MCL must not be released. Notch and medial compartment osteophytes are important to remove and the ACL and lateral compartment should be inspected. The lateral femoral condyle should be free of any articular cartilage lesions on the weight-bearing surface. If the

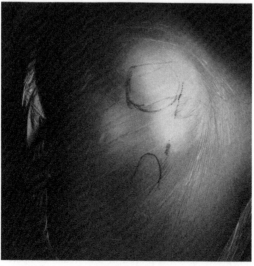

Fig. 7. The incision is made from the superomedial pole of the patella to the medial border of the tubercle.

ACL is deficient or there is more lateral articular cartilage damage than expected, the patient can be repositioned and the incision extended for a primary TKA.

The basic principle of implantation of the Oxford UKA is accurate balancing the flexion and extension gaps in the medial compartment. In order to accomplish a precise but minimal tibial resection, the Microplasty Instrumentation uses a series of sizing spoons that are intended to estimate the appropriate femoral component size and tension the MCL in flexion. Once the correct spoon has been chosen, the tibial guide is placed along the anteromedial tibia and connected to the spoon with a G clamp (**Fig. 8**). The tibial guide is then secured to the tibia with a pin and the medial tibial plateau can be resected with the typical vertical and horizontal saw cuts using special care to protect the MCL with the provided retractor (**Fig. 9**). The benefit of this spoon-based reference system is the accurate but minimalist approach to establishing a reliable flexion gap. Once the flexion gap is deemed sufficient, the femoral preparation can begin.

With the flexion gap established, the goal of femoral preparation is to fashion the medial femoral condyle for implantation of aspherical femoral component. This is accomplished by milling the medial femoral condyle into a round, spherical shape. The Microplasty Instrumentation uses a small intramedullary reference rod to position of the femoral component. Once the rod is inserted into a 5-mm opening hole at a point 1 cm anterior to the origin of the posterior cruciate ligament (PCL), the femoral drill guide is attached to this rod using a parallel intramedullary link (**Fig. 10**). This single step ensures that the femoral component is in the appropriate amount of flexion and rotation. Because the link is hinged, the linked femoral guide can be moved medially or laterally to ensure that the component is in the central one-third of the condyle. With the femoral drill guide in the correct position, a 4-mm anterior hole and 6-mm posterior hole is made in the distal medial femoral condyle (**Fig. 11**). Using a retractor to protect the MCL, the posterior condyle is then resected using a captured posterior resection guide that fits into these two holes.

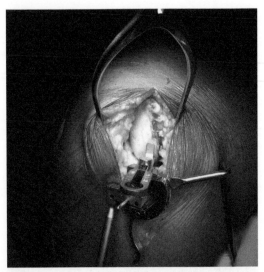

Fig. 8. Once the appropriate spoon is placed in the medial compartment to tension the MCL, it is linked to the tibial guide with the G clamp. This setup allows an accurate and minimalist tibial resection.

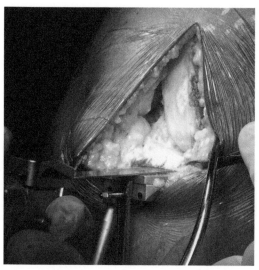

Fig. 9. Be sure to protect the MCL during the horizontal tibial cut.

The medial femoral condyle is made spherical using a specially designed mill (**Fig. 12**). The mill is cannulated and fits over various spigots that are inserted into the larger 6-mm femoral hole. The 0 spigot is used first to make the condyle a spherical shape to accept a spherical femoral trial. There is no distal bone removed with the first 0 spigot milling.

With the tibial and femoral trial components in place, the gaps are checked using feeler gauges of different thicknesses. The flexion gap should be measured with the

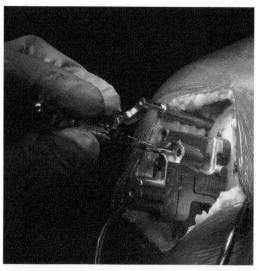

Fig. 10. After advancing the femoral intramedullary rod, the femoral drill guide is attached to the rod using the hinged link. This technique sets the component rotation and flexion, and allows the surgeon to position the drill guide on the middle third of the condyle.

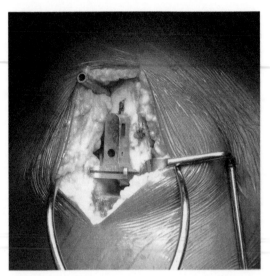

Fig. 11. Be sure to protect the MCL during the horizontal posterior condyle cut.

knee in 100 to 110° of flexion with slight valgus pressure and the extension gap should be measured in 15 to 20° of flexion with slight valgus pressure. The feeler gauge must be removed between gap checking because the MCL may be damaged if the knee is extended with a feeler gauge too large for the tight extension gap.

During the first evaluation of the gaps, it is common to have a flexion gap of 3 to 4 mm and an extension gap of 0 mm, or an extension gap too tight even for placing a gauge. The feeler gauge should move in and out of the compartment easily and have 1 mm of play without being able to tilt the gauge. If the flexion gap is too tight

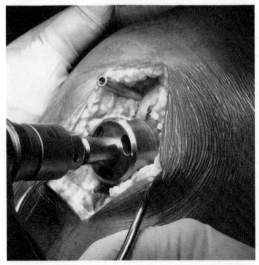

Fig. 12. After placing the 0 spigot, the condyle is made spherical using the appropriately sized femoral mill.

for a 3-mm gauge, more tibia needs to be resected because the thinnest bearing available is 3 mm.

Once the initial gap measurements are made, the distal femur is milled to balance the extension gap to the flexion gap. For example, if the flexion gap measures 3 mm and the extension gap measures 1 mm, then 2 mm of distal bone must be removed with the mill to achieve a balanced extension gap of 3 mm. In this scenario, this is accomplished by milling over the 2 spigot.

The most common reason for dislocation of the mobile bearing is impingement by posterior osteophytes or failure to remove enough bone around the anterior flange of the femoral component. The Microplasty Instrumentation has additional steps intended to remove bone in areas that could potentially impinge on the bearing. An anti-impingement guide is used to remove any posterior osteophytes or excessive anterior bone that would abut the bearing at terminal flexion and full extension (**Fig. 13**).

With the gaps now balanced and the potential sources of impingement addressed, a final trial is performed with a trial bearing rather than the feeler gauges (**Fig. 14A**). This trial bearing is symmetric and does not have the anatomic features of the bearing (see **Fig. 14B**). Without these anatomic qualities, the trial bearing may rotate slightly more than the anatomic bearing. Regardless, the trial bearing is intended to evaluate for residual bearing impingement, tracking, and insertion.

The bony surfaces are prepared with pulsatile lavage and drill holes for cement interdigitation. The tibial component is cemented first and it is critical to play close attention for cement fragments that may be left in the posterior recess of the medial compartment. If these fragments are left behind, they may irritate the remainder of the knee joint and cause a painful hemarthrosis. With both components in place, the components should be compressed with the appropriately sized feeler gauge at 45° of knee flexion and the cement allowed to harden. Once the cement has cured, the anatomic bearing can be placed and wound closure can begin. A cementless Oxford UKA is available in Europe but is not available in the United States at this time.

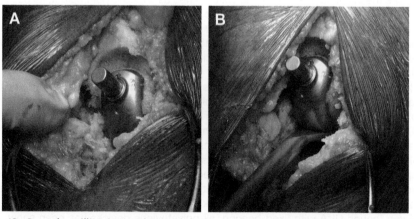

Fig. 13. Once the milling is complete and the knee is balanced in flexion and extension, the anti-impingement guide is used to resect a small amount of anterior bone using a specially designed mill (*A*) and has a posterior slot to remove any posterior osteophytes (*B*). This step is critical in removing the sources of impingement that can adversely affect bearing tracking.

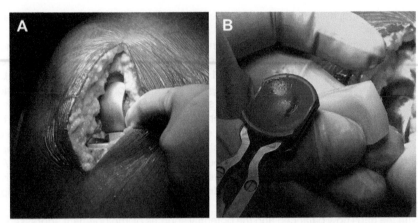

Fig. 14. The tracking and stability of the bearing are checked with the universal trial bearing (*A*). In contrast, the polyethylene bearing is side specific, with an elongated lateral border that improves tracking along the rail and prevents rotation (*B*).

The type of wound closure and use of a drain is surgeon preference. Patients are allowed weight bearing as tolerated but should use a knee immobilizer for 24 hours if the primary anesthesia is a femoral nerve block. Most Oxford UKA can be performed as an outpatient or 23-hour observation status. Most surgeons use physical therapy; however, many patients do not need therapy for as long as a typical patient having TKA. Although the incidence of deep vein thrombosis and pulmonary embolism after UKA is low compared with TKA, it is recommended that surgeons use their same strategy of prophylaxis in patients having UKA as in patients having TKA.[2]

RESULTS

Despite the initial poor results of the Oxford knee as a bicondylar implant, its use as a medial UKA for anteromedial osteoarthritis has seen outstanding long-term success. The Oxford designers published a 10-year survivorship of 98% with no failures secondary to polyethylene wear, tibial loosening, or patellofemoral disease.[5] In this series, the most common reason for the rare incidence of revision was progression of the arthritis to the lateral compartment.[5]

In an independent center outside the designing surgeons group, Svard and Price[6,7] maintained a meticulous and impressive follow-up of their series of Oxford UKAs with no patients lost to follow-up for more than 20 years. He published his survivorship at 10 and 20 years. The cumulative survivorship at 10 and 20 years were 95% and 91%, respectively.[6,7] The reasons for failure in this large series tended to be bimodal. Early failures within 2 years of implantation were secondary to bearing dislocation and infection, whereas later failures tended to be secondary to progression of lateral arthrosis and tibial side loosening. Again, no patients were revised secondary to the progression of patellofemoral disease or anterior knee pain.[6,7]

Even though UKA with fixed-bearing, all-polyethylene devices has been shown to have a poor survivorship in obese patients, obesity has not been a cause of early failure in an Oxford UKA series.[19,20] In the recent series by Murray and colleagues,[20] there was no significant difference in survivorship or objective knee score in any of the obese groups in the study. The change in functional score between before and after surgery was greatest for the most obese patients, indicating significant improvement in function after UKA.

In spite of these clinical outcome studies challenging the dogma of obesity and patellofemoral disease as contraindicators for UKA, ACL deficiency remains a contraindication to UKA. Multiple series of fixed-bearing UKA and one of Goodfellow and colleagues' initial Oxford series all cite ACL deficiency as a primary cause of UKA failure.[22–24] There have been multiple reports of successful Oxford UKA in combination with simultaneous ACL reconstruction but the long-term outcome has yet to be determined.[25,26] The combined procedure is technically challenging and currently considered an off-label use of the Oxford UKA in the United States.

Even with the notable long-term success of the Oxford UKA, perhaps the most impressive quality of the UKA is its safety profile compared with TKA.[2] Morris and colleagues[2] published on the postoperative morbidity and mortality after 1000 consecutive Oxford UKAs. There were no fatal pulmonary emboli and only 1 symptomatic deep vein thrombosis. The combined cardiac complication rate following UKA is lower than published rates for TKA. There were no deaths in the 90-day postoperative period, whereas the 90-day mortality following TKA has been documented to be 0.3% to 0.7%. In addition, infection following UKA was 0.1% compared with documented postoperative sepsis of 0.25% to 2.5% in TKA.

SURGICAL PEARLS

Most surgeons are comfortable with performing a TKA and understand the concepts of gap balancing. In contrast, many surgeons are uncomfortable with performing a UKA and consider it a more difficult surgery because of the unfamiliarity. However, like any procedure that a surgeon adopts, there is a learning curve. The Oxford UKA comprises the same basic concepts of the gap-balanced TKA coupled with greater forgiveness secondary to the spherical shape of the femoral component and improved accuracy with the Microplasty Instrumentation.

A detailed bullet-point list of pearls follows that may help the surgeon in early use of the Oxford UKA.

Preoperative evaluation
- Teach your staff how to perform a high-quality valgus stress radiograph on all varus knees with bone-on-bone arthritis (see **Figs. 2E** and **4**). The knee is bent 20° over a bolster and the x-ray beam should be angled 10° and aimed at the joint line.[10]
- Carefully evaluate the tibia on the lateral radiograph for posteromedial wear, which typically represents chronic ACL insufficiency.[12]
- A varus stress may help reveal bone-on-bone disease in cases with narrowing on the anteroposterior (AP) image (**Fig. 15**)
- Do not perform a UKA on a patient without bone-on-bone disease because the outcomes are unpredictable.[27]
- Patients with a contracted MCL do not correct with valgus stress and are better suited for TKA.

Surgical approach
- Start with a slightly longer incision than described and shorten it over time.
- Extend the arthrotomy into the vastus medialis. This allows the retinaculum to fall medially and enhances exposure of the MFC.
- Do not release the MCL when exposing the anteromedial tibia.
- Remove enough fat pad to easily see the ACL and lateral compartment.

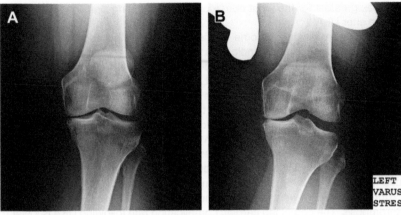

Fig. 15. (A, B) When there is obvious narrowing on the AP film, the varus stress film can be helpful in exposing bone-on-bone disease, which is important because the Oxford UKA is not suitable for patients with partial-thickness cartilage loss.

- If there is articular cartilage damage on the weight-bearing portion of the lateral femoral condyle, conversion to TKA is recommended.
- There may be an ulcer on the medial edge of the lateral femoral condyle near the notch that looks like an articular cartilage lesion. This ulcer is secondary to impingement against the tibial spine when the knee is in varus and is typically not weight bearing. This can be ignored.[10]
- If the ACL is deficient, conversion to TKA is recommended.

Tibial preparation
- Always protect the MCL. If the MCL is damaged, conversion to TKA is recommended.
- Remove the small anvil osteophyte in front of the ACL. Failure to do so may limit extension after surgery.
- The goal tibial slope is 7° and this is built into the tibial guide.
- Do not perforate the posterior cortex with the vertical saw cut because this may increase the risk of periprosthetic fracture.
- Remove all retractors when checking the gaps with the feeler gauges because the retractors falsely tension the MCL and make the gap seem too small.
- If the femoral drill guide does not fit in the flexion gap after making the tibial cut, the gap is too tight and more tibial resection is necessary.
- Do not remove the medial or posteromedial tibial osteophytes. The MCL may be damaged when attempting to remove these osteophytes.

Femoral preparation
- Remove the medial femoral osteophytes with a rongeur or osteotome but protect the MCL.
- Removed the notch osteophytes that impinge on the ACL.
- The starting hole for the intramedullary rod is more anterior than it seems.
- If the rod does not enter the canal by hand, check the trajectory and redrill.
- Do not use a mallet to advance the rod because it may perforate the cortex.
- Make sure the femoral drill guide is in the middle one-third of the condyle.
- Protect the MCL during the posterior femoral cut.

- Make sure there is no soft tissue in the teeth of the mill while reaming.
- Ream carefully in cases of AVN (**Fig. 5**). It is also essential to curette all dead bone and allow for ample cement interdigitation into the defect.
- If additional milling is needed after the first balancing attempt is made, do not use the mallet to seat the next spigot, because this may eliminate the reference point and result in overmilling.

Gap balancing
- Remember the gap balancing rules that apply for TKA.
- Check the flexion gap at 100 to 110° of flexion.
- Check the extension gap at 15 to 20° of flexion.
- Always remove the retractors when checking your gaps.
- Do not put in a bearing that is too tight because this may result in persistent postoperative tenderness along the medial tibia and MCL.

Oxford implantation
- Perform an adequate lavage of the bony surfaces.[28]
- Be careful to remove all pieces of the extruded cement because they can act as painful loose bodies if not removed.
- Compress the implant using the appropriate feeler gauge at 45° of knee flexion.

SUMMARY

With the societal push toward less invasive surgeries, rapid recovery, and return to a more active lifestyle, the UKA is an important tool for every orthopedic surgeon who treats osteoarthritis of the knee. In addition, the inherent safety profile of the UKA compared with TKA should be remembered when the TKA is referred to as the gold standard for the surgical treatment of end-stage osteoarthritis. In addition, the Oxford UKA seems to be ideally suited for use as an outpatient procedure that reduces cost and improves patient and surgeon satisfaction. There are many patients with varus osteoarthritis who are candidates for this less invasive option and clinicians owe it to their patients to investigate these options with appropriate preoperative evaluation and consideration regardless of their own tendencies and surgical skill sets.

The Oxford UKA and other designs have improved considerably over the past decade. These improvements in design, instrumentation, and outcomes make the UKA a powerful tool for all orthopedists. It is especially useful for those surgeons with a predominantly sports medicine practice, who are most likely to see those active patients with unicompartmental disease for which a TKA would be significantly limiting. Considering the lack of substantial polyethylene wear in the Oxford UKA mobile-bearing design, it is in these active sports medicine patients that the Oxford's benefits might be most evident.

REFERENCES

1. Romanowski MR, Repicci JA. Minimally invasive unicondylar arthroplasty: eight-year follow-up. J Knee Surg 2002;15(1):17–22.
2. Morris MJ, Molli RG, Berend KR, et al. Mortality and perioperative complications after unicompartmental knee arthroplasty. Knee 2012;20:218–20.
3. Berend KR, Lombardi AV Jr, Mallory TH. Rapid recovery protocol for perioperative care of total hip and total knee arthroplasty patients. Surg Technol Int 2004;13:239–47.

4. Patil S, Colwell CW Jr, Ezzet KA, et al. Can normal knee kinematics be restored with unicompartmental knee replacement? J Bone Joint Surg Am 2005;87(2): 332–8.
5. Murray DW, Goodfellow JW, O'Connor JJ. The Oxford medial unicompartmental arthroplasty: a ten-year survival study. J Bone Joint Surg Br 1998;80(6):983–9.
6. Svärd UC, Price AJ. Oxford medial unicompartmental knee arthroplasty: a survival analysis of an independent series. J Bone Joint Surg Br 2001;83(2):191–4.
7. Price AJ, Svard U. A second decade lifetable survival analysis of the Oxford unicompartmental knee arthroplasty. Clin Orthop Relat Res 2011;469(1):174–9.
8. Lindstrand A, Stenström A. Polyethylene wear of the PCA unicompartmental knee prospective 5 (4–8) year study of 120 arthrosis knees. Acta Orthop Scand 1992; 63(3):260–2.
9. Price AJ, Short A, Kellett C, et al. Ten-year in vivo wear measurement of a fully congruent mobile bearing unicompartmental knee arthroplasty. J Bone Joint Surg Br 2005;87(11):1493–7.
10. Goodfellow J, O'Connor J, Dodd C, et al. Unicompartmental arthroplasty with the Oxford knee. Oxford (United Kingdom): Oxford University Press; 2006. p. 1–67.
11. Goodfellow JW, O'Connor J. Clinical results of the Oxford knee surface arthroplasty of the tibiofemoral joint with a meniscal bearing prosthesis. Clin Orthop Relat Res 1986;205:21–42.
12. White SH, Ludkowski PF, Goodfellow JW. Anteromedial osteoarthritis of the knee. J Bone Joint Surg Br 1991;73(4):582–6.
13. Kozinn SC, Marx C, Scott RD. Unicompartmental knee arthroplasty a 4.5-6-year follow-up study with a metal-backed tibial component. J Arthroplasty 1989;4: S1–10.
14. Pandit H, Jenkins C, Gill HS, et al. Unnecessary contraindications for mobile-bearing unicompartmental knee replacement. J Bone Joint Surg Br 2011;93(5): 622–8.
15. Berend KR, Lombardi AV Jr, Adams JB. Obesity, young age, patellofemoral disease, and anterior knee pain: identifying the unicondylar arthroplasty patient in the United States. Orthopedics 2007;30:19–23.
16. Berend KR, Lombardi AV Jr, Morris MJ, et al. Does preoperative patellofemoral joint state affect medial unicompartmental arthroplasty survival? Orthopedics 2011;34(9):494–6.
17. Beard DJ, Pandit H, Ostlere S, et al. Pre-operative clinical and radiological assessment of the patellofemoral joint in unicompartmental knee replacement and its influence on outcome. J Bone Joint Surg Br 2007;89(12):1602–7.
18. Ingale PA, Hadden WA. A review of mobile bearing unicompartmental knee in patients aged 80 years or older and comparison with younger groups. J Arthroplasty 2013;28(2):262–7.
19. Berend KR, Lombardi AV Jr, Mallory TH, et al. Early failure of minimally invasive unicompartmental knee arthroplasty is associated with obesity. Clin Orthop Relat Res 2005;440:60–6.
20. Murray DW, Pandit H, Weston-Simons JS, et al. Does body mass index affect the outcome of unicompartmental knee replacement? Knee 2012. PubMed PMID: 23110877.
21. Bruni D, Iacono F, Raspugli G, et al. Is unicompartmental arthroplasty an acceptable option for spontaneous osteonecrosis of the knee? Clin Orthop Relat Res 2012;470(5):1442–51.
22. Deschamps G, Lapeyre B. Rupture of the anterior cruciate ligament: a frequently unrecognized cause of failure of unicompartmental knee prostheses. Apropos of

a series of 79 Lotus prostheses with a follow-up of more than 5 years. Rev Chir Orthop Reparatrice Appar Mot 1987;73(7):544–51.

23. Goodfellow JW, Kershaw CJ, Benson MK, et al. The Oxford Knee for unicompartmental osteoarthritis the first 103 cases. J Bone Joint Surg Br 1988;70(5): 692–701.

24. Swank M, Stulberg SD, Jiganti J, et al. The natural history of unicompartmental arthroplasty: an eight-year follow-up study with survivorship analysis. Clin Orthop Relat Res 1993;286:130–42.

25. Pandit H, Beard DJ, Jenkins C, et al. Combined anterior cruciate reconstruction and Oxford unicompartmental knee arthroplasty. J Bone Joint Surg Br 2006; 88(7):887–92.

26. Weston-Simons JS, Pandit H, Jenkins C, et al. Outcome of combined unicompartmental knee replacement and combined or sequential anterior cruciate ligament reconstruction: a study of 52 cases with mean follow-up of five years. J Bone Joint Surg Br 2012;94(9):1216–20.

27. Niinimäki TT, Murray DW, Partanen J, et al. Unicompartmental knee arthroplasties implanted for osteoarthritis with partial loss of joint space have high re-operation rates. Knee 2011;18(6):432–5.

28. Seeger JB, Jaeger S, Bitsch RG, et al. The effect of bone lavage on femoral cement penetration and interface temperature during Oxford unicompartmental knee arthroplasty with cement. J Bone Joint Surg Am 2013;95(1):48–53.

Robotic-assisted Unicompartmental Knee Arthroplasty: The MAKO Experience

Martin Roche, MD

KEYWORDS

- Unicompartmental knee arthroplasty • Robotic Assistance • MakoPlasty • Haptics

KEY POINTS

- This new robotic procedure provides comprehensive, 3-dimensional planning of partial knee components, including soft tissue balancing, followed by accurate resection of the femur and the tibia. This preparation allows for precise placement and alignment of the components.
- Patients have shown significant improvements in their postoperative function in every functional measurement, including more normal knee kinematics.
- The introduction of new procedures and technologies in medicine is routinely fraught with issues associated with learning curves and unknown potential complications.
- Because the specific objectives of this novel technology are to optimize surgical procedures to provide more safe and reliable outcomes, the favorable results seen to date prove this technology to be a significant improvement in the surgical technique of partial knee arthroplasty.

INTRODUCTION

In the late 1990s, Repicci and Eberle introduced a unicompartmental knee procedure using an inlay tibial component termed "minimally invasive surgery" (**Fig. 1**).[1–9] This procedure resulted in earlier mobilization, shorter inpatient stay, and shorter length of rehabilitation than had been observed for the conventional surgical approach. However, concerns were raised about loss of accuracy with minimally invasive techniques. With minimally invasive procedures, visualization is reduced leading to potential errors in implant placement, limb alignment, cement technique, and bone preparation (**Fig. 2**).[10,11]

The introduction of technology to improve accuracy of unicompartmental outcomes began with navigation. Jenny and colleagues[12] reported on a series of 60 patients who underwent navigated minimally invasive unicompartmental knee arthroplasty (UKA) and 60 patients who underwent navigated larger incision UKA. These authors cited

Holy Cross Orthopedic Institute 5597 N. Dixie Highway Fort Lauderdale, Florida 33334
E-mail address: Martin.roche@holy-cross.com

Clin Sports Med 33 (2014) 123–132
http://dx.doi.org/10.1016/j.csm.2013.08.007
0278-5919/14/$ – see front matter © 2014 Elsevier Inc. All rights reserved.

Surgical Errors: Key Points to Consider

Surgical Errors are fully in the surgeons' control and have a prominent effect on implant survival. A surgeon must familiarize himself with the system of choice and perform a consistent amount of surgeries to achieve consistent outcomes. Unicompartmental Knee Replacement (UKR)s are very unforgiving to technical errors, which often lead to early postoperative failures.

Common Errors

- Overcorrection of alignment
- Flexion-extension instability
- Not achieving cortical rim coverage with the tibial tray/ or allowing overhang of components
- Patellar arthritis (grade 4) or instability
- Inset tibial poly tray may subside
- Poor cement technique
- Anterior placed femoral component

Poor visualization can lead to

- Over/under resection of tibia
- Over/undercorrection of limb alignment

Implant placement

- Tibia—under coverage of cortex, overhang
- Anterior Cruciate Ligament (ACL) injury
- Excessive slope
- Mal-rotation—internal rotation-external rotation (IR-ER) of implants
- Patellar impingement
- Cement retention
- Pin site fracture
- Retained osteophytes

---

the advantages of reduced surgical trauma, reliability, and safety obtained with the navigated minimally invasive procedure, whereas radiographic accuracy of implantation was the same for both minimally invasive and larger incision navigation techniques.

Justin Cobb first introduced robotic assistance in 2000 using the Acrobot robot to improve the accuracy of implant positioning during UKA.

Cobb and colleagues[13] first reported a prospective comparison of a tactile-guided robot-assisted UKA and conventional UKA performed with manual instrumentation. Their robotic system used static referencing that required rigid intraoperative fixation of the femur and tibia to a stereotactic frame. The primary outcome measurement was the angle of the tibiofemoral alignment in the coronal plane, measured by computed tomography (CT). Implant position errors relative to the planned position averaged 1.1 mm and 2.5° with robotic assistance compared with 2.2 mm and 5.5° conventionally along any axis. Overall tibiofemoral coronal plane alignment was within 2° for every case performed with robotic assistance. Only 40% of conventional surgery achieved this level of accuracy.

In 2006, MAKO Surgical Corporation obtained US Food and Drug Administration clearance to begin the first implantation of medial UKAs using a haptic-controlled passive robotic arm. This system allows an accurate surgical preparation of the

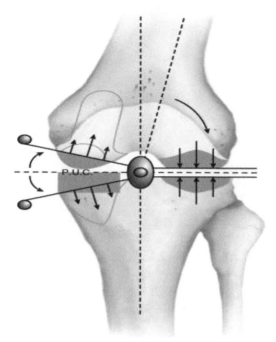

Fig. 1. The potential angular and rotation issues are depicted in unicompartmental implant placement.

specific patients' diseased knee compartment in one or multiple compartments, sparing healthy tissue in the undiseased compartments. This allows the surgeon to tailor the surgical procedure to the patient's arthritic and kinematic needs (**Fig. 3**). Addressing the medial, lateral, and patellofemoral joint in an individual, or modular manner, can be planned preoperatively and refined intraoperatively as the patient's knee kinematics and the disease pathology requires.

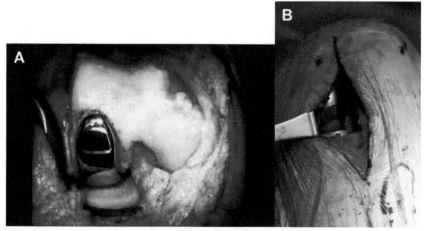

Fig. 2. Comparison of incision both approaches for (A) standard open and (B) minimally invasive implantation of UKA.

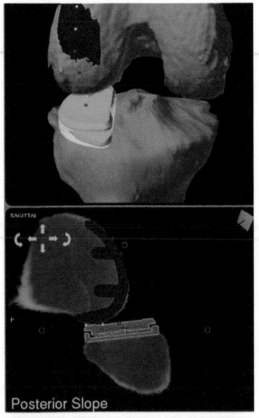

Fig. 3. The Patient's kinematic profile is evaluate on the computer screen through a full range of motion prior to burring.

Modular implants allowed inlay tibial or onlay tibial components to be used, with an anatomic femoral and trochlear implant. The implant design was based on CT-based parameters of more than 100 healthy and diseased knees. The femoral and patellofemoral components are created from a single, continuous surface. The inner geometries are contoured to allow bony preparation using a 6-mm burr. The femoral component allows deep flexion and has angled pegs to improve implant stability. The patellar component used in bicompartmental knee arthroplasty is a dome-shaped all polyethylene 3-pegged design, not pictured (**Fig. 4**).

The integration of robotic-arm assistance allows a surgeon to have a controlled, highly accurate system that is be integrated into the present surgical workflow. The enabling technology in this robotic platform was the development of haptics. Haptics is the science of applying touch (tactile) sensation and control to interaction with computer applications (**Fig. 5**). The evolution of this technology into the orthopedic arena was enabled by the ability of the surgeon to obtain an accurate reproducible surgical result in all 6 degrees of freedom (3 translational and 3 rotational), which the human eye cannot reproduce to the same level of precision.

This system uses optical motion capture technology to dynamically track marker arrays fixed to the robotic arm, femur, and tibia, allowing the surgeon to freely adjust limb position and orientation during tactile-guided bone cutting. This

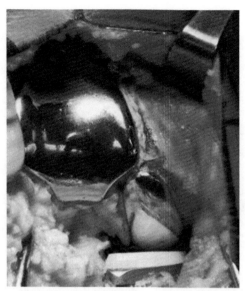

Fig. 4. The modular implants showing a medial UKR and Trochlear implant in a bicompartmental knee replacement.

robotic-assisted platform enables the surgeon to use a preoperative computer-assisted planning system and a high-speed burr controlled by a tactile guidance system intraoperatively, thus eliminating the need for conventional instrumentation.

There are several systems in place throughout the procedure to ensure accuracy is achieved. Tibial and femoral checkpoints must be verified before each section of bone is prepared. At any point throughout the procedure, the robotic-arm and mechanical burr tip can be removed from the surgical zone and a tracker probe can be used to visualize accuracy and cuts directly on the patient's CT scan (**Fig. 6**).

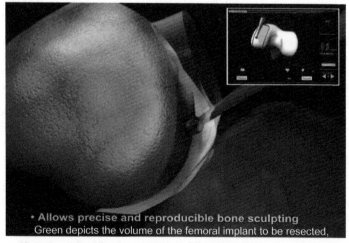

Fig. 5. Virtual bone resection shows the RIO burr in a 3-dimensional virtual haptic safe zone. Burr is only active for cutting when burr tip is within haptic safe zone.

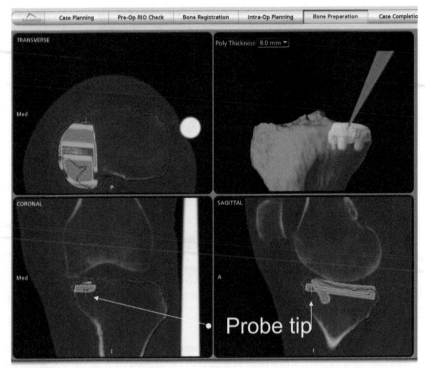

Fig. 6. Screen capture from software shows how probe confirms planned depth of cut on CT view.

During burring, the surgeon receives visual, auditory, and haptic feedback to ensure adherence to the surgical plan. Visual feedback is depicted on the user interface module. Green bone on the screen indicates bone to be removed; white bone on the screen indicates the surgeon has removed the necessary bone, and red bone on the screen depicts when the planned implant placement threshold has been penetrated up to 0.5 mm (**Fig. 7**). If penetration occurs beyond 0.5 mm, the burr tip shuts off. When approaching the implant boundaries, a surgeon receives auditory feedback with a beeping noise. Haptic feedback refers to the tactile sensation of the arm physically resisting a surgeon's applied force when the haptic boundary is approached. Boundaries are specified to match the implant shape, size, and placement based on intraoperative planning. Cement tolerances are included in boundaries.

Roche and Coon have reported the accuracy of this system in accurate implant placement. Coon and colleagues[14] radiographically compared 44 manually implanted UKAs to 33 robotically implanted. The accuracy of implant positioning with robotic-arm assistance was improved by a factor of 2.8 in the sagittal plane and an average root-mean-square (RMS) error of 3.2° in the coronal plane as compared with the accuracy of manual, jig-based instrumented UKAs.[14] Roche and colleagues[15] radiographically measured postoperative implant placement accuracy on a series of 43 UKA patients. Average RMS errors were 1.9° in the coronal plane and 1.7° in the sagittal plane. More recently, Roche and colleagues published 3-dimensional accuracy results from postoperative CT scan taken for 20 of the first 50 patients to ever receive the procedure. For this study, all average RMS errors were found to be

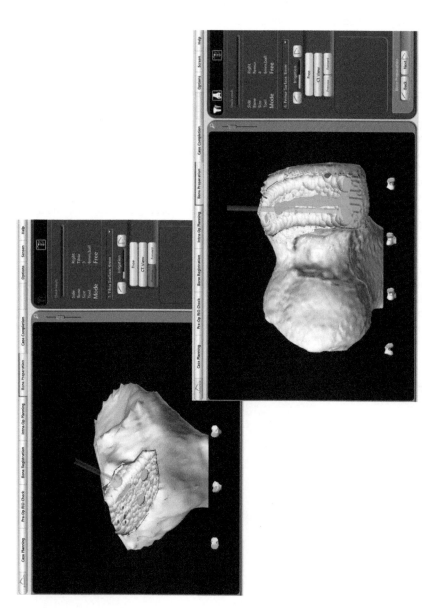

Fig. 7. Screen captures taken during burring of tibia (*left*) and femur (*right*) show bone being resected. Green bone represents bone still to be burred. Red bone indicates any cut that is made outside of 0.5 mm from the plane. The burr will shut off beyond 1 mm of planned resection.

within 1.6 mm and 3.0° in all directions. These patients demonstrated good or excellent outcomes including average Knee Society Scores (KSS) at 3 years of 88 and 75 for knee and function, respectively. At 6 weeks, the range of motion (ROM) improved from a preoperative value of 119° to 126° of flexion and was maintained at 125° out to 3 years postoperatively.[16]

Radiographs reveal precise, repeatable, and accurate implant placement (**Fig. 8**). These images confirm this historically difficult surgery can be performed with minimally invasive approaches, supplemented with a robotic-arm to achieve predictable reproducible results.

The proposed benefits of a robotic-assisted platform include the ability to resurface only the painful degenerative knee surfaces and retain healthy structures, which leads to improved kinematics, stability, and proprioception. Watanabe and colleagues[17] reported the kinematics for a series of 15 knees to receive partial knee replacement whereby all knees showed normal posterior lateral condylar translation while kneeling and performing a step activity. These findings more closely represented normal knee kinematics than TKA patients that underwent the same test procedure.

Although the robotic arm ensures accurate implant placement, many additional factors are required for a surgeon to achieve a successful surgical outcome. The ability to perform the predicted surgical plan consistently and precisely is related to proper implant sizing and positioning specific to the patients' anatomy, optimizing the tension/balance of the collateral and cruciate ligaments through the entire ROM, actualizing smooth implant-cartilage transitions through cartilage mapping software, and the ability to minimize bone resection and tissue injury during surgery with haptic boundaries.

Through a minimal incision, optimized implant placement and soft tissue balancing enables a rapid rehabilitation program that enables patients to return to activities of daily living or resume work with minimal recovery times.

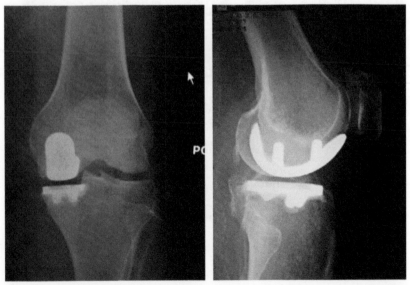

Fig. 8. Anteroposterior and lateral postoperative radiographs show precise placement of robotic-arm–assisted UKA.

CLINICAL OUTCOMES

Roche and colleagues[18] reported outcomes for the first 73 patients to receive robotic-arm–assisted UKA. There were 42 men in the group and patient's average age was 71 ± 10 years. The average body mass index for patients was 29 with 38% of the population considered obese. At 2 years postoperatively, patients saw an increased average ROM of 129° of flexion compared with a preoperative ROM of 123°. Postoperative KSS also increased from 43.8 preoperatively to 96.8 postoperatively for knee scores and 63.9 preoperatively to 80 postoperatively for their function scores.

Coon and colleagues[19] reported patient outcomes for 36 of their initial robotic-arm–assisted UKAs and compared those results with the 45 cases performed just before the introduction of robotic technology with manual instruments using a mini-invasive technique. They saw no significant difference in average knee society score (KSS), average change in KSS, or Marmor rating at postoperative follow-up. These findings suggest results are comparable with accepted technique and show there was not a detectible learning curve effect manifest in clinical outcomes with this new technology.

SUMMARY

This new robotic procedure provides comprehensive, 3-dimensional planning of partial knee components, including soft tissue balancing, followed by accurate resection of the femur and the tibia. This preparation allows for precise placement and alignment of the components. Patients have shown significant improvements in the postoperative function in every functional measurement, including more normal knee kinematics. The introduction of new procedures and technologies in medicine is routinely fraught with issues associated with learning curves and unknown potential complications. Because the specific objectives of this novel technology are to optimize surgical procedures to provide more safe and reliable outcomes, the favorable results seen to date prove this technology to be a significant improvement in the surgical technique of partial knee arthroplasty.

REFERENCES

1. Aleto TJ, Berend ME, Ritter MA, et al. Early failure of unicompartmental knee arthroplasty leading to revision. J Arthroplasty 2008;23(2):159–63.
2. Collier MB, Eickmann TH, Sukezaki F, et al. Patient, implant, and alignment factors associated with revision of medial compartment unicondylar arthroplasty. J Arthroplasty 2006;21(6 Suppl 2):108–15.
3. Ridgeway SR, McAuley JP, Ammeen DJ, et al. The effect of alignment of the knee on the outcome of unicompartmental knee replacement. J Bone Joint Surg Br 2002;84(3):351–5.
4. Collier MB, Engh CA Jr, McAuley JP, et al. Factors associated with the loss of thickness of polyethylene tibial bearings after knee arthroplasty. J Bone Joint Surg Am 2007;89(6):1306–14.
5. Arno S, Maffei D, Walker PS, et al. Retrospective analysis of total knee arthroplasty cases for visual, histological, and clinical eligibility of unicompartmental knee arthroplasties. J Arthroplasty 2011;26(8):1396–403.
6. Moro-oka TA, Muenchinger M, Canciani JP, et al. Comparing in vivo kinematics of anterior cruciate-retaining and posterior cruciate-retaining total knee arthroplasty. Knee Surg Sports Traumatol Arthrosc 2007;15(1):93–9.
7. Hall VL, Hardwick M, Reden L, et al. Unicompartmental knee arthroplasty (alias uni-knee). An overview with nursing implications. Orthop Nurs 2004;23(3): 163–71 [quiz: 172–3].

8. Banks SA, Fregly BJ, Boniforti F, et al. Comparing in vivo kinematics of unicondylar and bi-unicondylar knee replacements. Knee Surg Sports Traumatol Arthrosc 2005;13(7):551–6.

9. Repicci JA, Eberle RW. Minimally invasive surgical technique for unicondylar knee arthroplasty. J South Orthop Assoc 1999;8(1):20–7 [discussion: 27].

10. Müller PE, Pellengahr C, Witt M, et al. Influence of minimally invasive surgery on implant positioning and the functional outcome for medial unicompartmental knee arthroplasty. J Arthroplasty 2004;19(3):296–301.

11. Fisher DA, Watts M, Davis KE. Implant position in knee surgery: a comparison of minimally invasive, open unicompartmental, and total knee arthroplasty. J Arthroplasty 2003;18(7 Suppl 1):2–8.

12. Jenny JY, Ciobanu E, Boeri C. The rationale for navigated minimally invasive unicompartmental knee replacement. Clin Orthop Relat Res 2007;463:58–62.

13. Cobb J, Henckel J, Gomes P, et al. Hands-on robotic unicompartmental knee replacement: a prospective, randomised controlled study of the acrobot system. J Bone Joint Surg Br 2006;88(2):188–97.

14. Coon TM, Driscoll MD, Conditt MA. Robotically assisted UKA is more accurate than manually instrumented UKA. J Bone Joint Surg Br 2010;92(Supp I):157.

15. Roche MW, Augustin D, Conditt MA. Accuracy of robotically assisted UKA. J Bone Joint Surg Br 2010;92(Supp I):127.

16. Dunbar NJ, Roche MW, Park BH, et al. Accuracy of dynamic tactile-guided unicompartmental knee arthroplasty. J Arthroplasty 2012;27(5):803–8.e1.

17. Watanabe T, Kreuzer S, Leffers K, et al. Is Cruciate-Ligament Functionality Retained In Partial and Multicompartmental Knee Arthroplasty? in Orthopaedic Research Society Annual Meeting. San Francisco, CA, 2012.

18. Roche MW, Horowitz S, Conditt MA. Four year outcomes of robotically guided UKA. in 23rd Annual Congress of ISTA. Dubai, UAE, 2010.

19. Coon T, Driscoll M, Conditt MA. Early Clinical Success of Novel Tactile Guided UKA Technique. in 21st Congress of the ISTA. Sacramento, CA, 2008.

Patient-Specific Instrumentation and Return to Activities After Unicondylar Knee Arthroplasty

Joel L. Boyd, MD, Chad A. Kurtenbach, MD, Robby S. Sikka, MD*

KEYWORDS

- Unicompartmental knee arthroplasty • Arthroplasty • Osteoarthritis • Osteotomy
- Knee

KEY POINTS

- Unicompartmental knee arthroplasty (UKA) is an excellent surgical option for isolated medial or lateral unicompartmental osteoarthritis (OA). Initial studies were discouraging, but recent studies report greater than 85% survivorship at 10 years, with approximately 90% of patients reporting good to excellent subjective and objective outcomes.
- When comparing function and return to recreational activity, UKA is at least equivalent to high tibial osteotomy (HTO).
- Advantages of UKA versus total knee arthroplasty (TKA) include preserved bone stock, decreased recovery time, more normal gait kinematics, improved quadriceps function, and increased knee flexion.
- UKA revision to TKA may be technically easier than TKA revision, but reported outcomes are more similar to a revision TKA than to a primary TKA. New implants and improved surgical techniques, however, lead to less bone loss and may make conversion to TKA easier in the future.
- There are a variety of implant designs and surgical techniques for UKA. Custom cutting blocks have been designed to aid in preoperative planning and to streamline the surgical technique. The authors' early results with custom block technology suggest fewer malpositioned implants, decreased surgical time, and excellent short-term functional results.

UNICOMPARTMENTAL KNEE ARTHROPLASTY

This information is designed to help physicians and health care providers understand

- Indications and contraindications for UKA
- Expected outcomes for patients undergoing primary UKA and conversion to TKA
- Potential complications of UKA
- Discuss patient specific instrumentation and its impact on technique and preoperative planning

---

TRIA Orthopaedic Center, 8100 Northland Drive, Bloomington, MN 55416, USA
* Corresponding author.
E-mail address: Robby.sikka@tria.com

Clin Sports Med 33 (2014) 133–148
http://dx.doi.org/10.1016/j.csm.2013.08.003
0278-5919/14/$ – see front matter © 2014 Elsevier Inc. All rights reserved.

INTRODUCTION

Original UKA implants were often placed without the benefit of reliable instrumentation and guide systems. Many UKA systems now have instrumentation that is equivalent to TKA systems.[1–13] These advances have improved the ability to place better-designed devices in more predictable positions. Taking that a step further, custom cutting blocks have been introduced by several companies in hopes of further improving the accuracy of the technique and subsequent implant position. These custom cutting guides are created to match individual patient anatomy using preoperative advanced imaging (MRI or CT). These cutting blocks may improve preoperative assessment of the deformity, streamline the surgical technique, and allow for more accurate implant placement.

UKA implants are currently manufactured in fixed-bearing and mobile-bearing designs. The fixed-bearing model may be all metal backed or all polyethylene. With a fixed-bearing design, in particular one that has a metal-backed tibial component, loosening is rare, reoperations for wear are infrequent, and survivorship is high. The mobile-bearing design has two important potential benefits: decreased rate of wear and decreased stress at the interface between the cemented implant and bone that could translate into a lower rate of prosthotic loosening. This has generated interest in mobile-bearing designs, but studies to date have failed to demonstrate superior results using the mobile-bearing implants.[6,14] Additionally, the surgical technique is more demanding when using mobile-bearing implants and the risk of bearing dislocation is a legitimate concern.

The current surgical treatment options for unicompartmental OA include HTO, UKA, and TKA. There is a significant amount of overlap in the indications for these treatment options. HTO is often used in young, active patients that are expected to live longer than the expected survival of the prosthesis. Patients undergoing TKA are typically older and have more advanced OA of the knee. UKA has become a popular option for surgeons due to improved implant design and reproducible surgical technique. When compared with TKA, typical inpatient stays are shorter, recovery from surgery is often quicker, knee kinematics are closer to the native knee, and complication rates are thought to be lower. When compared with HTO, UKA shows comparable results with regards to function and return to activity. An HTO is still a good procedure for young patients, but it should be noted that in patients with grade IV cartilage damage with involvement of more than one-third of the condylar surface or an osteochondritis dissecans lesion of more than 5 mm deep, osteotomy alone may not be sufficient to restore adequate function to the knee. A cartilage restoration procedure in conjunction with the HTO may lead to improved outcomes in certain situations. There are still unpredictability and longevity concerns, however, with current cartilage procedures. UKA should be considered an option in this scenario, and the authors think that this procedure can result in good to excellent functional outcomes in the majority of patients. Most patients are able to return to a variety of different sporting activities.

INDICATIONS

UKA is typically considered in younger and more active patients but also is considered in older sedentary patients with noninflammatory OA confined to a single tibiofemoral compartment (**Fig. 1**). To consider UKA, there should be minimal clinical patellofemoral or contralateral compartment symptoms. Knee range of motion (ROM) should include at least 100° of flexion and any fixed flexion contracture should be less than 10°. Historically, additional selection criteria included a maximum of 10° of varus or 5° of valgus deviation from the mechanical axis. The varus/valgus deformity needs

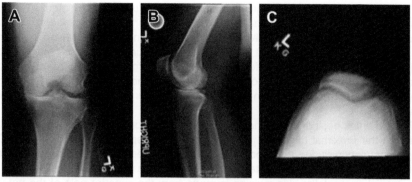

Fig. 1. (*A*) Anteroposterior, (*B*) lateral, and (*C*) sunrise radiographs showing isolated medial compartment OA.

to be correctable on physical examination because the UKA cannot be used to correct extra-articular malalignment. Mediolateral subluxation or other significant ligamentous insufficiency is a contraindication to UKA. An intact anterior cruciate ligament (ACL) has been advocated as an absolute criteria for UKA, but recent studies and author experience suggest that decreasing the tibial slope can successfully be used to accommodate for an insufficient ACL. Morbid obesity has been described as a relative contraindication with the most commonly used body mass index cutoff of 35.

Additional indications and contraindications are described in **Table 1**.

SURGICAL TECHNIQUE

The surgical goals of UKA are to replace damaged articular surfaces, restore limb alignment, and create a mechanical axis close to neutral to avoid overloading the contralateral compartment. Several different UKA guide systems can be used (intramedullary, extramedullary, spacer block, custom cutting blocks, and so forth) to ensure accurate osseous cuts and proper implant position. After surgical reconstruction, the joint line should be parallel to the floor and perpendicular to the mechanical axis. The femoral and tibial implants should be oriented perpendicular to the mechanical axis. The corresponding author prefers to use MRI-based patient-specific instrumentation (PSI), and the technique discussed illustrates the use of these custom cutting guides.

When using the PSI system, a preoperative MRI is performed following a specific protocol that determines limb alignment and individual patient anatomy. Once the

Table 1
Indications and contraindications for unicompartmental knee arthroplasty

Indications	Contraindications
Unicompartmental OA	Inflammatory arthritis
Young and/or active patient	Bicompartmental or tricompartmental arthritis
Minimal bone loss <5 mm	Fixed flexion deficit >10°
Flexion >100°	>10° Varus or >5° valgus deformity
	Ligamentous laxity
	Previous meniscectomy in contralateral compartment
	ACL deficiency[a]
	Morbid obesity[a]

[a] Relative contraindication.

MRI has been performed, a surgical plan is developed using a computerized model. This plan is made available on-line to the surgeon performing the operation. The surgeon has the ability to preoperatively visualize patient anatomy to develop a customized surgical plan for each patient (**Fig. 2**). It allows the surgeon to modify the plan, and adjustments can be made to the following parameters: implant selection, implant size, resection depth, femoral rotation, varus/valgus, flexion/extension, and posterior slope. After the preoperative plan is approved by the surgeon, the 3-D cutting blocks are created.

The patient is positioned supine on a conventional operating table. A tourniquet is used on the proximal thigh and the leg should be prepped free to allow full ROM and manipulation during the procedure. The technique discussed is based on performing a medial UKA, but the steps are the same for a lateral UKA.

A medial parapatellar skin incision is made from the superior pole of the patella, extending 2 cm to 4 cm distal to the joint line adjacent to the tibial tubercle. The joint is entered through a medial parapatellar arthrotomy and most surgeons elect to evert the patella to allow for thorough inspection of all three compartments. After the knee joint is exposed, the fat pat is removed as necessary to facilitate visualization. A minimal soft tissue medial release is carried out by dissecting subperiosteally along the joint line back toward, but not into, the medial collateral ligament. Overcorrection should be avoided and an undercorrection of 2° to 3° of the mechanical axis is thought to be desirable and leads to long-term survivorship.

In the authors' surgical technique, the preference is to address the tibia first. Osteophytes are not removed when using the PSI system because the custom cutting blocks are created to accommodate existing osteophytes for a secure fit. Osteophytes should be removed if using other guide systems. The anterior half of the meniscus is removed to expose the medial tibial plateau and additional soft tissue is removed as needed to allow proper placement of the tibial guide. Externally rotating the tibia can help facilitate exposure to the medial tibia. The tibial cutting guide is positioned on the medial plateau and should conform anatomically to the tibia (**Fig. 3**A-C). Ensure proper fit by verifying contact through the windows of the guide and around the

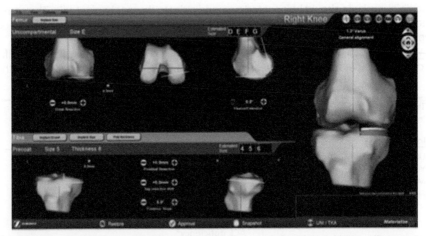

Fig. 2. Illustration of computer software used to create PSI for planned UKA. Allows preoperative planning for the following: implant size of femur/tibia, femoral rotation, tibial rotation, resection depth, varus/valgus, flexion/extension, and posterior slope.

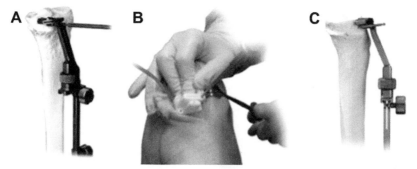

Fig. 3. (*A*) The standard tibial guide is shown in the sagittal and coronal planes. (*B, C*) The PSI tibial cut guide is positioned on the medial plateau and should conform anatomically to the tibia.

periphery. The guide is held in place using headless pins and headed screws. Avoid overtightening of the headed screws because this may torque the guide and lead to an inaccurate tibial cut.

The alignment rod is then placed into the guide to ensure accurate alignment (**Fig. 4**). The alignment rod should be parallel to the tibial crest and be in line with the center of the ankle. If the alignment is inaccurate, reposition the guide and recheck with the alignment rod. When using the PSI system, the amount of tibial resection and posterior slope can be adjusted preoperatively and built into the custom blocks. The depth of tibial cut should be approximately 2 mm to 4 mm and a posterior slope of 5° to 7° is standard.

The proximal tibial cut is made using a narrow oscillating saw (ensure that the medial collateral ligament is protected with a retractor). If using the PSI system, there is a predetermined depth of the cut and this can be marked on the saw to avoid penetration of the posterior soft tissue structures. On completion of the proximal cut, the saggital cut is made using a reciprocating saw. Cut along the edge of the ACL down to, but not beyond, the intended level of the transverse cut. The cutting guide is then removed and the medial plateau is excised using an osteotome.

Attention is turned to the femur. With the knee in approximately 45° of flexion, the patella is moved laterally to allow for placement of the femoral resection guide. The femoral cut guide is positioned on the femur and should create a stable and unique fit (**Fig. 5**). The knee is then brought into extension and the tension guide (2 mm or 3 mm) is placed between the femoral guide and the cut surface of the tibia to preliminarily check the flexion/extension gap prior to cutting the femur. The tension guide serves as the appropriate amount of space (2–3 mm) that should be between the

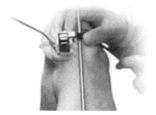

Fig. 4. The alignment rod is then placed into the guide to ensure accurate alignment.

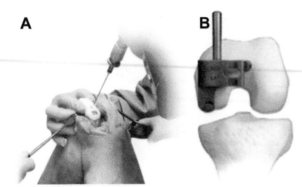

Fig. 5. (*A*) With the knee in approximately 45° of flexion, the PSI femoral cut guide is positioned on the femur. (*B*) The standard femoral resection guide.

implants during the final trial. To verify tension, the knee should come into full extension and there should be stability to varus and valgus stress. After appropriate tension is verified, the femoral cutting guide is secured with headed screws. It is recommended to tighten the lateral screw first to minimize movement of the guide. It is important to again avoid overtightening of the screws to prevent placing torque on the guide. The knee is brought into flexion and positioning of the guide is confirmed. The knee is then brought into extension and the distal femoral cut is made using an oscillating saw (**Fig. 6**). The PSI report includes a saw blade excursion depth and can be used to avoid deep penetration of the saw. Remove the femoral guide and the distal femoral bone resection. After removing the resection guide, ensure that the cut surface of the distal femur is completely flat. If necessary, modify the cut so that it is flat. This is important because future cuts depend on this initial femoral cut.

The flexion/extension gap should be checked at this point. Flexion/extension gap spacers come in 8 mm, 10 mm, 12 mm, and 14 mm. Start with an 8-mm spacer and adjustments can be made accordingly. If the gap is too tight, more distal femur or proximal tibia needs to be cut. If the gap is too loose, upsize the spacer and recheck. Standard UKA balancing rules are used for an asymmetric flexion/extension gap.

After verifying the flexion/extension gap, the knee is brought into flexion and the femur is sized. There should be 2 mm to 3 mm of exposed bone at the anterior edge of the guide when sizing is appropriate (**Figs. 7** and **8**). The guide is held in place by

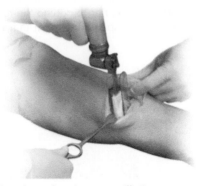

Fig. 6. The distal femoral cut is made using an oscillating saw.

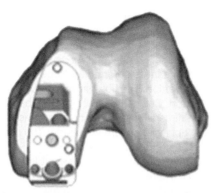

Fig. 7. The femoral finishing guide is aligned with the predrilled hole at the proximal aspect of the guide.

placing a headed screw into the femoral finishing guide. The femoral rotation is then confirmed by ensuring that the posterior surface of the femoral guide is parallel to the tibial cut. There should be exposed bone on both the medial and lateral aspects of the femoral guide to avoid overhang. When position is confirmed, the femoral

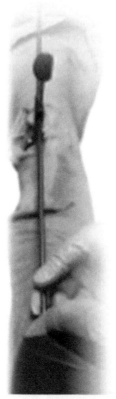

Fig. 8. The femoral finishing guide is aligned with the predrilled hole at the proximal aspect of the guide.

finishing guide is secured to the femur and the remaining femoral cuts are completed. The femoral guide is removed and any remaining prominences, osteophytes, and uncut bone are resected to ensure that the cut surfaces are flat.

At this point of the procedure, alignment should be verified with a spacer block and alignment rod. Once the alignment is determined to be accurate, attention is turned back to the tibia for final preparation. The tibial sizer is used to verify the recommended implant size from the PSI report. Select the tibial sizer that best fits in both the anterior/posterior and medial/lateral dimensions. Place the appropriately sized tibial baseplate onto the cut surface of the tibia and secure with a pin. The peg holes are then drilled and the baseplate is left in place for trial reduction.

The femoral, tibial, and polyethylene trials are assembled and inserted. The knee is tested for ROM and stability. There should only be 2 mm to 3 mm of space between the components under varus and valgus stress in a neutral position. After trial reduction, the femoral prosthesis is cemented, followed by cementing of the tibial implant. The trial polyethylene is inserted and the knee is extended, allowing for the cement to set. Once the cement is cured, adjustments to the size of the polyethylene can be made and the final poly implant is selected and placed into the tibial component. Thorough irrigation of the knee is done using a pulse lavage and care is taken to tightly close the arthrotomy site. Skin is closed in standard fashion and sterile bandages are applied.

The authors do not routinely use a drain for UKA, but some surgeons may elect to place a drain for 24 hours. Routine antibiotics are used for 24 hours postoperatively. Mechanical venous thrombolism (VTE) prophylaxis is started on admission and pharmacologic VTE prophylaxis is started on postoperative day 1 and is typically continued for 2 to 4 weeks. Patients can safely be weight bearing as tolerated with a walker or crutches immediately. Physical therapy is continued on an inpatient and outpatient basis after a similar protocol for TKA. Radiographs should be taken on an annual basis to follow progression of adjacent compartment arthritic changes as well as any wear or change in the status of the implant (**Fig. 9**).

OUTCOMES

Outcomes from studies are summarized in **Tables 2** and **3**.[10,14–24] These tables summarize articles with greater than 10-year follow-up (**Table 3**) as well as recent articles

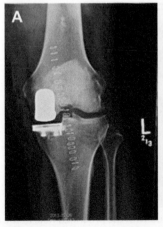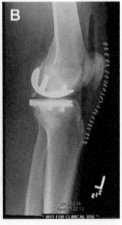

Fig. 9. (*A*, *B*) Standard anteroposterior and lateral postoperative radiographs.

Table 2
Studies of unicompartmental knee arthroplasty with minimum 10-year follow-up

Author, Year	Number of Patients	Minimum Length of Follow-up (y) (Mean)	Prosthesis Design	Number of Failures	Reasons for Failure			
					Patellofemoral Compartment	Adjacent Compartment	Aseptic Loosening	Other[a]
Marmor,[16] 1988	60	10 (11)	Marmor	21 (35%)	2%	3%	18%	12%
Weale & Newman,[10] 1994	42	12 (N/A)	St. George Sled	5 (12%)	N/A	N/A	N/A	N/A
Cartier et al,[15] 1996	60	10 (12)	Marmor	9 (15%)	0	3%	2%	10%
Squire et al,[22] 1999	140	15 (17)	Marmor	14 (10%)	0	5%	4%	1%
Svard & Price,[24] 2001	124	10 (13)	Oxford	6 (5%)	0	0	2%	3%
Hernigou & Deschamps,[18] 2002	99	10 (14)	Lotus	22 (22%)	1%	3%	17%	1%
Khan et al,[21] 2004	30	10 (N/A)	St. George Sled	2 (7%)	0	0	3%	3%
Price et al,[14] 2005	114	10 (N/A)	Oxford	24 (21%)	0	9%	5%	7%
Berger et al,[17] 2005	62	10 (N/A)	Miller-Galante	2 (3%)	3%	0	0	0
O'Rourke et al,[20] 2005	136	21 (N/A)	Marmor	19 (14%)	N/A	7%	6%	1%
Steele et al,[23] 2006	203	10 (15)	St. George Sled	16 (8%)	0.5%	3%	0.5%	4%
Newman et al,[19] 2009	24	15 (15)	St. George Sled	4 (17%)	0	8%	4%	4%

Abbreviation: N/A, not available.
[a] Other causes include infection, arthrofibrosis, fracture, recurrent hemarthrosis, and unexplained pain that could not be attributed to disease progression or loosening.

Table 3
Selected studies published since 2010

Author, Year	Number of Patients	Effective Follow-up Percentage	Length of Follow-up	Prosthesis	Complications	Outcomes
Pandit et al,[6] 2011	1000	55%	5.6 y	Oxford III	2.9% Reoperation rate 2 Revisions requiring stemmed replacements and 17 conversions to TKA; 6 open reductions for bearing dislocations and 3 secondary lateral UKAs and 1 tibial revision	Mean Oxford knee score was 41.3 (SD 7.2), the mean American Knee Society Objective Score 86.4 (SD 13.4), mean Tegner activity scale score 2.8 (SD 1.1). Mean maximum flexion was 130°. Overall survival rate at 10 y was 96%.
Lecuire et al,[5] 2013	65 Knees	64%	11 y (Mean)	ALPINA Cementless	11 (17%) Revision procedures. 1 for Early knee degeneration on RA patient, 1 for OA in adjacent compartment, 1 for unexplained pain, 1 for late ACL rupture, 3 for polyethylene insert fracture, 4 due to severe poly wear.	Mean IKS improved from 119.3 ± 16.8 to 171.4 ± 25.3 (P<.0001); 89% rated good to excellent; knee flexion improved from 120.5° to 127.3° (P<.01). Overall survival rate 88%; survival rate was 94% when revision due to implant mechanical failure used as endpoint.

Clement et al,[2] 2012	49 Knees	100%	7.2 y (Mean)	Oxford III	2 Patients passed away prior to 5-y follow-up (unrelated to knee surgery). 4 Early failures: 1 failure due to AVN of lateral femoral condyle, 3 with anterior knee pain without signs of OA.	Cumulative survival was 91.2%
Heyse et al,[3] 2012	223 Knees	100%	10.8	Genesis/ Accuris	15 Implant failures were recorded (6.7%) with average time to revision was 76.7 mo.	KSS knee score 94.3, KSS function score 94.9. Implant survival 94.3%. Survivorship for entire cohort 93.5% at 10 y and 86.3% at 15 y.
Foran et al,[4] 2013	19 Knees in 16 patients (original study was 62 knees in 51 patients)	31%	15 y	Miller-Galante/ Zimmer	Four of 62 knees were revised to TKA at a mean of 144 mo: 2 due to adjacent compartment progression, 1 as a result of poly disengagement and metallosis, and 1 for pain of unclear etiology. 34 Patients lost to death and 1 lost to follow-up	15-Year survivorship was 93% and 20-y survivorship was 90%.

Abbreviations: AVN, avascular necrosis; IKS, international knee score; KSS, knee society score; RA, rheumatoid arthritis.

from post-2010 (see **Table 3**).[2–6] The authors think that the recent articles highlight the newer implants available as well as many of the long-term studies that have recently been published. Because most current studies have shown survival rates of 85% to 90% at 10 to 15 years of follow-up, the authors think there is a need to emphasize potential complications and their relative rates.[25] There is a relative dearth of articles reporting on outcomes of PSI implants. Understanding what factors in this population may have an impact on return to sport is something that requires further research as is which patients may have benefited from HTO.

Examination of complication rates for UKA versus HTO tend to show a greater rate of wound complications and deep vein thrombosis (DVT) after HTO.[7,9,10] Thus, confounding factors predisposing to wound healing problems, such as diabetes, should be taken into account before HTO. The increased rate of DVT may be due to longer weight-bearing restrictions in the HTO population leading to less early postoperative motion in the HTO population.[7,9,10] Postoperative stiffness requiring manipulation under anesthesia tends to occur more often in UKA and may be related to less preoperative motion in these patients or possibly age differences in the patient populations because HTO is more common in younger patients.[10] Complication rates after TKA and UKA are similar and do not show any significant trends.[13,26]

Outcomes comparing HTO and UKA have shown slightly superior outcomes in the HTO cohorts in most studies; however, these findings have not been statistically significant.[7,9,10] Weale and Newman reported higher knee function scores in the UKA cohort and noted that their findings were statistically significant.[26] Thus, it is likely that good to excellent outcomes can be expected in both groups and that risk factors and desired activity level should be used to determine which surgical option may result in the best outcomes. Studies comparing UKA and TKA for unicompartmental arthritis have not shown statistically significant differences between the two techniques. Good to excellent results can be expected in 85% to 90% of patients at 10 to 15 years' follow-up in both groups and other factors should be considered, including desired activity level, potential for subsequent procedures, and comorbidities.[13,26]

Naal and colleagues[11] reported on 83 patients who underwent UKA and evaluated participation in sports at a mean of 18 months postoperatively. They noted that prior to surgery, 77 of 83 patients were engaged in an average of 5.0 sports and recreational disciplines; postoperatively, 73 (88%) participated in an average of 3.1 different sports, resulting in a return to activity rate of 95%. The most common activities after surgery were hiking, cycling, and swimming. Several high-impact activities as well as the winter disciplines of downhill and cross-country skiing had a significant decrease in participating patients. A majority of the patients (90.3%) stated that surgery had maintained or improved their ability to participate in sports or recreational activities.[11] Pietschmann and colleagues[12] also reported on return to sports after UKA. They noted patients in the active group were significantly younger than the patients in the inactive group ($P<.05$). A majority of patients (80.1%) returned to their level of sports activity after UKA surgery and concluded that use of the Oxford III implant could result in a high rate of return to sport.[12]

COMPLICATIONS

A complete list of potential complications is described in **Box 1**. As with TKR, UKA does also has the possibility of polyethylene wear and is more common with incongruity between the femoral component and the tibial insert. As longer follow-up studies have been performed, a distinction has been made between early and late failures (those occurring after 10 years), with late failures typically due to polyethylene wear.

Box 1
Potential complications
Technique error[a]
Infection
DVT or pulmonary embolism
Bone loss
Progression of contralateral compartment
Polyethylene wear
Bearing dislocation
Aseptic loosening
Mechanical failure
Periprosthetic fracture
[a] See text for more detailed discussion of common surgical technique errors.

This was addressed by the development of the Oxford unicompartmental knee replacement with a spherical femoral surface and a flat tibial surface, providing a mobile-bearing design and more normal kinematics. The bearing can behave like the meniscus by moving forward and backward during knee motion, and this is the most commonly used UKA in England with excellent survivorship at 15 years. It generally is recommended that the minimum safe thickness of polyethylene to use is 6 mm. With the Oxford prosthesis, a bearing of appropriate thickness is chosen intraoperatively to correctly tension the ligaments of the knee. The range of thicknesses available (measured at the thinnest part of the bearing) starts at 3.5 mm and increases in 1-mm intervals.[2,6,25,27–29]

Bearing dislocation is a common cause of failure in mobile-bearing UKA. It is typically due to an imbalance in the flexion and extension gaps. Lateral mobile UKA is more prone to bearing dislocation because of the increased natural mobility of the lateral side of the joint. Moreover, wear of the posterior condyle is possible because the surgical technique used cannot easily define the flexion gap joint line. Fixed-bearing designs thus may be easier to insert but have a higher incidence of bearing failure in the medium and long term. Fixed-bearing implants, such as the Tornier HLS (Montbonnot-Saint-Martin, France), have a flat all polyethylene tibial component, and a polycentric femoral component. This particular implant has shown excellent 10-year survivorship (>90%). Survivorship analysis based on component loosening and revision showed a 99% survival for the meniscal-bearing implant and 93% survival for the fixed-bearing implant at 11 years. Yet, although the 10-year outcomes are similar for the Oxford *unicompartmental knee replacement* and the Tornier HLS, this may not be the case at 20-years when polyethylene wear may become apparent in the fixed-bearing design. Despite this, because a fixed-bearing cannot dislocate, this design may have advantages for surgeons with a lower volume practice.[2,6,25,27–29]

The experience of the surgeon may play an important role in the survival of the prosthesis. Robertsson and colleagues[30] reported higher revision rates in surgeons who performed fewer than 23 UKAs. One of the most common surgeon-associated complications is progression of arthritis in the lateral compartment, which can be caused by overcorrection of the deformity. Kennedy and White[31] have shown that the best results occur when alignment is slightly undercorrected. The reason why knees are overcorrected is to achieve stability of the mobile bearing. There is a tendency to use the largest possible bearing, with the potential unintentional consequence of overcorrecting the knee into valgus alignment. The worst situation is represented when the varus is low with an over-reducibility of the deformity. Additionally, progression of OA changes may also be noted in the patellofemoral compartment as well, as described by Hernigou and Deschamps.[18]

Other complications may include overaggressive medial release, which may lead to medial collateral ligament injury affecting postoperative therapy and mobilization and also lead to instability or decreased ROM. Additionally, underappreciation of the tibial slope may lead to instability postoperatively. Hernigou and Deschamps[32] noted a significant linear relationship between anterior tibial translation (mean, 3.7 mm) and posterior tibial slope (mean, 4.3°) ($P<.01$). They suggested greater than 7° of posterior slope of the tibial implant should be avoided, particularly if the ACL is absent at the time of implantation.[32] An intact ACL, even when partly degenerated, was associated with the maintenance of normal anteroposterior stability of the knee for an average of 16 years after UKA.

FUTURE AREAS OF RESEARCH

Future research on UKA will likely continue to expand on the indications of this procedure. Return to sports activity in increasingly active 50- to 60-year-old patients will likely necessitate further evaluation. Development of improved implant materials may be required as patients have increasing demands and a strong desire to return to preoperative function. Although the current generation of implants has shown good outcomes for 15 to 20 years with minimal wear, perhaps the next generation of patients will have greater sporting demands or require UKA at a younger age, thereby testing the survival rates of the current generation of UKAs.

The authors think that studies should also be done on short-term and long-term outcomes of PSI implants. Because custom cutting blocks (**Fig. 10**) are created for individual patients, they are designed to streamline the surgical technique and ideally decrease technical errors. Further comparison of this generation of implants with earlier generations of implants and with TKA are needed to understand the implications of UKA.

Studies evaluating the cost-effectiveness of the current generation of PSI implants versus TKA or current UKA options will also help improve cost utilization as reimbursements continue to decline.

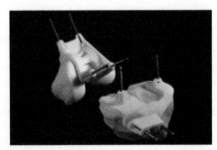

Fig. 10. Custom cutting blocks are created for each individual patient. They are designed to streamline the surgical technique and decrease technical errors.

REFERENCES

1. Riddle DL, Jiranek WA, McGlynn FJ. Yearly incidence of unicompartmental knee arthroplasty in the United States. J Arthroplasty 2008;23(3):408–12.
2. Clement ND, Duckworth AD, MacKenzie SP, et al. Medium-term results of Oxford phase-3 medial unicompartmental knee arthroplasty. J Orthop Surg (Hong Kong) 2012;20(2):157–61.
3. Heyse TJ, Khefacha A, Peersman G, et al. Survivorship of UKA in the middle-aged. Knee 2012;19(5):585–91.
4. Foran JR, Brown NM, Della Valle CJ, et al. Long-term survivorship and failure modes of unicompartmental knee arthroplasty. Clin Orthop Relat Res 2013; 471(1):102–8.
5. Lecuire F, Berard JB, Martres S. Minimum 10-year follow-up results of ALPINA cementless hydroxyapatite-coated anatomic unicompartmental knee arthroplasty. Eur J Orthop Surg Traumatol 2013. [Epub ahead of print].
6. Pandit H, Jenkins C, Gill HS, et al. Minimally invasive oxford phase 3 Unicompartmental knee replacement: results of 1000 cases. J Bone Joint Surg Br 2011;93(2): 198–204.
7. Borjesson M, Weidenhielm L, Mattsson E, et al. Gait and clinical measurements in patients with knee osteoarthritis after surgery: a prospective 5-year follow-up study. Knee 2005;12:121–7.
8. Ivarsson I, Myrnerts R, Gillquist J. High tibial osteotomy for medial osteoarthritis of the knee. A 5 to 7 and 11 year follow-up. J Bone Joint Surg Br 1990;72(2): 238–44.
9. Stukenborg-Colsman C, Wirth CJ, Lazovic D, et al. High tibial osteotomy versus unicompartmental joint replacement in unicompartmental knee joint osteoarthritis: 7-10-year follow-up prospective randomised study. Knee 2001;8(3):187–94.
10. Weale AE, Newman JH. Unicompartmental arthroplasty and high tibial osteotomy for osteoarthrosis of the knee. A comparative study with a 12- to 17-year follow-up period. Clin Orthop Relat Res 1994;(302):134–7.
11. Naal FD, Fischer M, Preuss A, et al. Return to sports and recreational activity after unicompartmental knee arthroplasty. Am J Sports Med 2007;35(10):1688–95.
12. Pietschmann MF, Wohlleb L, Weber P, et al. Sports activities after medial unicompartmental knee arthroplasty Oxford III-what can we expect? Int Orthop 2013; 37(1):31–7.
13. Cameron HU, Jung YB. A comparison of unicompartmental knee replacement with total knee replacement. Orthop Rev 1988;17(10):983–8.
14. Price AJ, Waite JC, Svard U. Long-term clinical results of the medial Oxford unicompartmental knee arthroplasty. Clin Orthop Relat Res 2005;435:171–80.
15. Cartier P, Sanouiller JL, Grelsamer RP. Unicompartmental knee arthroplasty surgery. 10-year minimum follow-up period. J Arthroplasty 1996;11:782–8.
16. Marmor L. Unicompartmental arthroplasty of the knee with a minimum ten-year follow-up period. Clin Orthop Relat Res 1988;228:171–7.
17. Berger RA, Meneghini RM, Jacobs JJ, et al. Results of unicompartmental knee arthroplasty at a minimum of ten years of follow-up. J Bone Joint Surg Am 2005;87:999–1006.
18. Hernigou P, Deschamps G. Patellar impingement following uni-compartmental arthroplasty. J Bone Joint Surg Am 2002;84:1132–7.
19. Newman J, Pydisetty RV, Ackroyd C, et al. Unicompartmental or total knee replacement: the 15-year results of a prospective random- ised controlled trial. J Bone Joint Surg Br 2009;91:52–7.

20. O'Rourke MR, Gardner JJ, Callaghan JJ, et al. The John Insall Award: unicompartmental knee replacement: a minimum twenty-one- year followup, end-result study. Clin Orthop Relat Res 2005;440:27–37.

21. Khan OH, Davies H, Newman JH, et al. Radiological changes ten years after St George Sled unicompartmental knee replacement. Knee 2004;11:403–7.

22. Squire MW, Callaghan JJ, Goetz DD, et al. Unicompartmental knee replacement. A minimum 15 year fol- lowup study. Clin Orthop Relat Res 1999;(367):61–72.

23. Steele RG, Hutabarat S, Evans RL, et al. Survivorship of the St George Sled medial unicompartmental knee replacement beyond ten years. J Bone Joint Surg Br 2006;88:1164–8.

24. Svard UC, Price AJ. Oxford medial unicompartmental knee arthroplasty. A survival analysis of an independent series. J Bone Joint Surg Br 2001;83:191–4.

25. Mercier N, Wimsey S, Saragaglia D. Long-term clinical results of the Oxford medial unicompartmental knee arthroplasty. Int Orthop 2010;34:1137–43.

26. Weale AE, Halabi OA, Jones PW, et al. Perceptions of outcomes after unicompartmental and total knee replacements. Clin Orthop Relat Res 2001;(382):143–53.

27. Kori NP, van Raay JJ, van Horn JJ. The Oxford phase III unicompartmental knee replacement in patients less than 60 years of age. Knee Surg Sports Traumatol Arthrosc 2007;15:356–60.

28. Lisowski LA, van den Bekerom MP, Pilot P, et al. Oxford Phase 3 unicompartmental knee arthroplasty: medium-term results of a minimally invasive surgical procedure. Knee Surg Sports Traumatol Arthrosc 2011;19:277–84.

29. Bruni D, Iacono F, Russo A, et al. Minimally invasive unicompartmental knee replacement: retrospective clinical and radiographic evaluation of 83 patients. Knee Surg Sports Traumatol Arthrosc 2010;18:710–7.

30. Robertsson O, Knutson K, Lewold S, et al. The routine of surgical management reduces failure after unicompartmental knee arthroplasty. J Bone Joint Surg Br 2001;83(1):45–9.

31. Kennedy WR, White RP. Unicompartmental arthroplasty of the knee. Postoperative alignment and its influence on overall results. Clin Orthop Relat Res 1987;(221):278–85.

32. Hernigou P, Deschamps G. Posterior slope of the tibial implant and the outcome of unicompartmental knee arthroplasty. J Bone Joint Surg Am 2004;86(3):506–11.

Outcomes and Complications of Unicondylar Arthroplasty

Andrew J. Riff, MD[a], Alexander P. Sah, MD[b],
Craig J. Della Valle, MD[a],*

KEYWORDS

- Unicompartmental knee arthroplasty • Patellofemoral compartment
- Lateral compartment • Medial compartment

KEY POINTS

- With careful attention to specific patient and anatomic indications, unicompartmental knee arthroplasty offers clinical results and survivability that are as good, or better, than total knee arthroplasty.
- Unicompartmental knee arthroplasty results in diminished perioperative morbidity compared with total knee arthroplasty.
- Unicompartmental knee arthroplasty can be converted to total knee arthroplasty with relative technical ease.
- Although not performed as frequently as medial unicompartmental knee arthroplasty, with a few specific technical alterations lateral unicompartmental knee offers a reliable option for management of isolated lateral compartmental arthritis.
- Unicompartmental knee arthroplasty is an alternative to total knee arthroplasty in appropriate selected patients and is not a "bridge" procedure.

INTRODUCTION

Unicompartmental knee arthroplasty (UKA) was initially introduced in the early 1960s as an alternative to total knee arthroplasty (TKA) for arthrosis limited to either the medial or lateral tibiofemoral compartment. Proponents of UKA cited its ease of implantation, minimal bone sacrifice, more natural-feeling knee, more normal gait, and ease of revision to TKA as rationale for selecting UKA over TKA. Nevertheless, a combination of poor prosthetic design and instrumentation and poor patient selection led to high rates of failure in early series.[1–6] As a result of high rates of failure, UKA was widely abandoned by the late 1980s. In the last 15 years, UKA has seen resurgence

[a] Section of Adult Reconstruction, Department of Orthopaedic Surgery, Rush University Medical Center, 1611 West Harrison, Suite 300, Chicago, IL 60612, USA; [b] Institute for Joint Restoration, Washington Hospital, 2000 Mowry Avenue, Fremont, CA 94538, USA
* Corresponding author.
E-mail address: craigdv@yahoo.com

Clin Sports Med 33 (2014) 149–160
http://dx.doi.org/10.1016/j.csm.2013.06.005
0278-5919/14/$ – see front matter © 2014 Elsevier Inc. All rights reserved.

as several studies have demonstrated that survivorship of UKA is comparable or superior with that of TKA in appropriately selected patients.

HISTORIC DURABILITY AND SURVIVORSHIP OF DESIGN

Modern UKA first developed in the 1960s with tibial hemiarthroplasty implants. Introduced in 1964, the MacIntosh prosthesis consisted of a single piece of cobalt-chrome that had a smooth concave superior surface and a flat serrated inferior surface. The McKeever prosthesis, developed around the same time, was a similar tibial metal-resurfacing prosthesis that included a T-shaped fin on the undersurface for additional fixation. Short and intermediate follow-up studies demonstrated good results in 70% to 80% of patients undergoing hemiarthroplasty.[1–3] More recently, Springer and colleagues[4] demonstrated a 50% revision rate of 26 knees treated with the McKeever prosthesis at average 8 years, with all being easily converted to either UKA or TKA. Remaining patients had good function at long-term follow-up (mean, 16.7 years). The McKeever tibial hemiarthroplasty was concluded to be a reasonable surgical option in patients who are not candidates for osteotomy or UKA.

In the late 1960s, UKA progressed to prostheses that resurfaced both the tibial and femoral surfaces, with the introduction of such implants as the polycentric knee, the St. Georg sled, and the Marmor. These prostheses were used in either a unicompartmental or bicompartmental manner depending on the extent of arthritic involvement. Initial reports were concerning because of high rates of early failure. Laskin[6] reported minimum 2-year follow-up data on 37 patients treated with the Marmor UKA. In the follow-up interval, eight patients (22%) required revision surgery and more than half of patients in the series experienced settling of the tibial component greater than 1 mm. Revisions were performed for progression of arthritis in the other tibiofemoral compartment (four patients); patellofemoral pain (two patients); severe unexplained knee pain (one patient); and loosening of the tibial components (one patient). Insall and Aglietti[5] reported 5- to 7-year follow-up results of 32 patients undergoing hemiarthroplasty in the early 1970s. Of 22 patients available for follow-up, 7 required revision surgery (32%) and only 8 experienced a good result.

By the end of the 1980s, more encouraging reports began to appear in the literature demonstrating results of UKA that were comparable with TKA and better than osteotomy in the appropriate patient population. Thornhill[7] reported excellent results in 92% of patients at 42-month follow-up. Capra and Fehring reviewed results from 52 patients undergoing UKA at 8.3-year follow-up and predicted survivorship of 93.75% at 10-years postarthroplasty, comparable with contemporary reports of TKA survivorship.[8] Kozinn and colleagues[9] reported good or excellent results in 92% of knees at a mean 5.5-year follow-up after UKA with a metal-backed tibial component. Ninety-two percent of the knees were rated as having a good or excellent result, and 94% had lasting relief of pain. There were no failures requiring revision. Heck and colleagues[10] demonstrated a 10-year survivorship rate of 91.4% in 294 patients undergoing UKA with the Marmor prosthesis at multiple centers. These promising reports were all tempered by caveats stressing proper patient selection with regard to patient-specific and anatomic factors.

MODERN UNICOMPARTMENTAL INDICATIONS

In light of increased emphasis on patient selection, Kozinn and Scott[11] outlined specific indications for UKA in 1989 with regard to patient age, weight, activity level, pain, range of motion, and angular deformity. In terms of patient-specific factors, they recommended that patients be more than 60 years old; have low demand for activity (neither extremely active nor perform heavy labor); weigh less than 180 pounds; and have minimal pain at rest. In terms of anatomic factors, they recommended that patients have at least a 90-degree arc of flexion; flexion contracture less than or equal to 5 degrees; minimal angular deformity (range, 10 degrees of varus deformity to 15 degrees of valgus deformity); and a passively correctable angular deformity (after osteophyte excision).

Although these indications provided a good starting point, Goodfellow and colleagues[12] suggested that some of these contraindications could be ignored for mobile-bearing UKA and that UKA should be indicated more based on pathoanatomy. Specifically, they supported UKA for patients with bone-on-bone degeneration of the medial compartment, an intact anterior cruciate ligament and medial collateral ligament, and retained cartilage in the lateral compartment; they coined this term "anteromedial arthritis." Pandit and colleagues[13] reviewed a series of 1000 UKAs of which 678 (68%) had at least one potential contraindication according to the guidelines of Kozinn and Scott's publication and 322 (32%) were thought to be "ideal" candidates. The series demonstrated that 10-year survival was 97% for those with potential contraindications and 93.6% in "ideal" patients.

With osteotomy becoming less common, UKA is more frequently used in the younger patient. Although durability in this younger population needs further evaluation, results thus far have been excellent. The lead author evaluated 85 medial UKAs in patients younger than age 55 at an average of 4 years postoperatively. Patients demonstrated exceptional Knee Society (95.1) and UCLA Activity (7.5) scores. Ten-year projected survival was 96.5%. Additionally, no patient demonstrated radiographic evidence of component loosening, osteolysis, or premature polyethylene wear. In terms of the older population, the elderly may particularly benefit from the less invasive surgery and less morbidity associated with UKA. Sah and colleagues[14] demonstrated remarkable durability of UKA implants in a series of UKA performed in 28 octogenarians between 1978 and 1990. At final follow-up, 24 of 25 patients had well-functioning replacements and also were outlived by their prosthesis. At this point, there is no set of universally accepted indications; however, all are used in unison as general guidelines.

MOBILE-BEARING UKA

In 1978, the Oxford mobile-bearing prosthesis was introduced by Goodfellow and O'Connor.[15] This system is composed of a highly congruent articulation between the femoral component and polyethylene coupled with a flat tibial tray on which the polyethylene rests. The large contact area (roughly 6 cm^2) of the femoral- and tibial-polythene interfaces results in lower polyethylene stresses and, in turn, extremely low wear measurements (0.01–0.03 mm/y).[16] The designers of the Oxford medial-compartment UKA demonstrated striking survivability of the system with a 98% cumulative prosthetic survival rate at 10 years. In another series, Price and colleagues[17] demonstrated comparable results with 94% survival of 420 medial UKAs at 15-year follow-up. Despite these good results, mobile-bearing implants come with a 1% to 2% risk of polyethylene dislocation, require an intact anterior cruciate ligament, and cannot be used in the lateral compartment secondary to a higher risk of bearing dislocation with the presently available design, although a new unique design that incorporates a domed tibial component may mitigate this problem. Gunther and colleagues[18] reported on 53 lateral Oxford UKAs at average 5-year follow-up and found that 75% were functioning well but 21% had failed, many of which related to dislocation.

ADVANTAGES OF UKA

If the indications outlined previously are observed, UKA offers distinct advantages over TKA: it requires less bony resection, results in less blood loss, allows a faster recovery, is associated with lower morbidity than TKA, can be relatively easily converted to TKA, preserves all of the knee ligaments, and results in better range of motion and probably a more normal-feeling knee.

In the 1990s, UKA garnered increased attention in the United States with the development of surgical techniques that facilitated implantation through a smaller incision. Repicci and Eberle[19] pioneered a surgical technique for UKA that is done through a smaller incision (3 in vs 8 in required for TKA) and uses bone preparation techniques that emphasize preservation of bone. Fisher and colleagues[20] retrospectively compared the results of 41 patients who underwent UKA with 50 patients who underwent TKA. They demonstrated that blood loss was significantly less for the UKA group, as was the need for blood transfusion. Additionally, narcotic use and length of hospital stay were also significantly less for the unicompartmental group. Brown and colleagues[21] also examined risk of perioperative morbidity by retrospectively reviewing results of 2235 primary TKA and 605 primary UKA at multiple centers. They demonstrated that UKA is associated with an overall lower risk of complication (4.3% vs 11%; P<.0001); need for postoperative blood transfusion (0.2% vs 1.6%; P = .036); admission to an intensive care unit (0.2% vs 1.4%; P = .049); and need for discharge to a rehabilitation facility (3.1% vs 18%; P<.0001). Although not statistically significant, they also observed a trend toward significance with regard to lower risks of deep periprosthetic joint infection (0.2% vs 0.8%; P = .21); readmission to the hospital (2.7% vs 4.2%; P = .079); venous thromboembolic events (0.64% vs 1%; P = .398); and reoperation (0.6% vs 1.4%; P = .32).

With the advent of minimally invasive techniques, UKA has also offered a more normal-feeling knee. Isaac and colleagues[22] demonstrated that UKA resulted in significantly greater improvements in dynamic proprioception than did TKA. Additionally, Patil and colleagues[23] performed and in vitro cadaver study that demonstrated that TKA rendered statistically significant changes from native tibial rotation during walking, whereas UKA resulted in no alteration in tibial rotation. These advantages, in conjunction with improving survivorship, promoted a reemergence of UKA in the late 1990s and early 2000s. Between 1998 and 2005, prevalence of UKA increased at a rate three times that of TKA.

LATERAL UKA

Isolated arthritis of the lateral compartment is less common than its medial counterpart. Despite the increase in popularity of UKA throughout the last 15 years, lateral compartment UKA still constitutes only 10% of UKAs performed.[24] In light of differences in anatomy, biomechanics, and wear patterns in the lateral compartment, unique considerations must be taken into account before performing lateral UKA. Mobile-bearing UKA is not recommended in the lateral compartment in light of the risk of bearing instability. However, fixed-bearing partial knee designs can have excellent success in the lateral compartment. Surgical considerations with lateral UKA begin with surgical approach and include component placement considerations. The surgical approach for placement of a lateral UKA can be executed through a lateral parapatellar approach. Disadvantages of this approach include less soft tissue on the lateral side for wound closure, a less familiar technique, and concerns of patellar avascular necrosis if a medial approach is performed for revision surgery. In light of these concerns, Sah and Scott[25] described a technique to use the medial parapatellar approach to safely perform lateral UKA; a key difference in the surgical approach is the necessity of not damaging the coronary ligament or medial meniscus when the medial arthrotomy is performed.

In addition to surgical approach, lateral UKA also requires technical considerations to prevent patellar impingement and to restore the screw-home mechanism.[24,26] The laxity of the lateral compartment can lead to a higher likelihood of overstuffing, which leads to medial compartment progression, and a careful assessment of soft tissue tension is required. Tibial internal rotation with increasing knee flexion requires a more internally rotated tibial component placement, which can be difficult to achieve, particularly if a lateral approach is used (**Fig. 1**). Because the patella tends to ride laterally in the trochlea, the risk of impingement of the patella against the femoral component is higher (**Fig. 2**), and proper downsizing of the femoral component is required to avoid patellar impingement (**Fig. 3**). Lastly, the femoral component should be shifted laterally to maximize tibiofemoral component congruency in extension. If appropriate modifications are made, lateral UKA can provide superb long-term results. Pennington and colleagues[26] reported a series of 29 lateral UKAs that were all in place and well functioning at an average of 12.4 years postoperatively. Similarly, Sah and Scott[25] also reported 100% survivability of 49 lateral UKA at an average 5.2-years follow-up.

PATELLOFEMORAL ARTHROPLASTY

Arthritis isolated to the patellofemoral joint is less common than arthritis isolated to either the medial or lateral compartment alone. Studies have shown that this arthritis pattern can be well treated with total knee replacement. Similar to the aforementioned

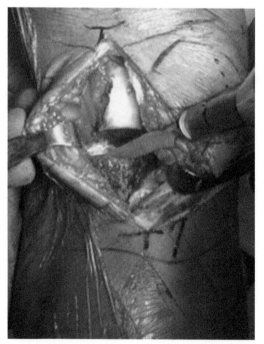

Fig. 1. Care is taken to make a tibial cut that permits internal rotation of the tibial component.

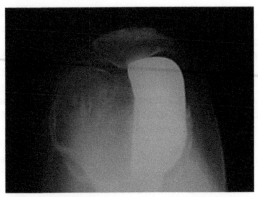

Fig. 2. Merchant radiograph demonstrating patellar impingement secondary to an oversized femoral component after lateral UKA.

benefits of UKA, patellofemoral replacement spares the cruciate ligaments and the remaining two compartments. Much like UKA at large, early generations of patellofemoral arthroplasty (PFA) were fraught with high rates of failure; however, more modern designs have been promising. First-generation designs failed primarily because of tracking problems, patellar catching, anterior knee pain, and arthritis progression in the tibiofemoral compartments.[27] Many of these problems were secondary to an overconstrained design resulting from a narrow trochlear implant that was deep and

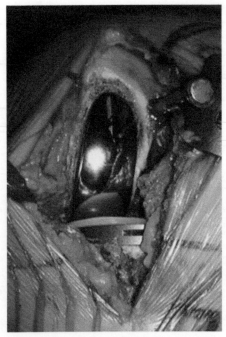

Fig. 3. The femoral component is intentionally undersized relative to the native femoral condyle to minimize the risk of patellar impingement.

unforgiving.[28] Nevertheless, recent series have demonstrated excellent results. Sisto and Sarin[29] reported 100% good or excellent outcomes and 100% survivability at a mean of 73-months follow-up in a series of 25 patients treated with a custom PFA. Dahm and colleagues[30] compared 23 PFAs with 22 TKAs and concluded that PFA renders a comparable clinical outcome at 29-months follow-up with less blood loss and perioperative morbidity. Still, two long-term follow-up series (mean, 16 and 17 years, respectively) revealed that evolution of tibiofemoral osteoarthritis is the most common reason for failure of PFA and that tibiofemoral osteoarthritis requiring conversion to TKA occurred in 21% and 18% of patients, respectively (**Fig. 4**).[31,32]

UKA VERSUS TKA

In addition to the aforementioned theoretical advantages of UKA, trials directly comparing UKA with TKA have demonstrated that UKA frequently outperforms TKA with regard to range of motion, patient satisfaction, knee scores, survivorship, and cost. Dalury and colleagues[33] compared outcomes of 23 patients who had undergone UKA on one side and TKA on the other. They demonstrated improved range of motion with the UKA compared with the TKA (123 ± 9 degrees vs 119.8 ± 7 degrees, respectively). Additionally, they found that of the 23 patients, 12 subjectively preferred the unicompartmental knee and the remainder had no preference. Newman and colleagues[34] randomized 102 knees to either St. Georg sled UKA or kinematic modular TKA. At 15-year follow-up, patients undergoing UKA demonstrated a higher likelihood of having an excellent Bristol knee score (71% for UKA compared with 53%) and a higher survivorship rate (90% for UKA compared with 79% for TKA). In a series of 200 arthritic knees requiring arthroplasty, Willis-Owen and colleagues[35] demonstrated that UKA rendered better functional scores than TKA (based on Total Knee Questionnaire scores); that medial and lateral UKA both rendered scores comparable with healthy age-matched knees; and that UKA offered a substantially lower cost than TKA (£1761 per knee).

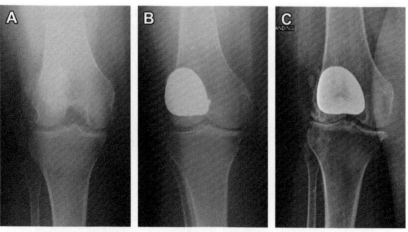

Fig. 4. (A) Preoperative radiograph of a patient with PFA demonstrating well-preserved medial and lateral tibiofemoral joint. (B) Postoperative radiograph 6 weeks status post-PFA demonstrating preservation of medial and lateral tibiofemoral joint space. (C) Postoperative radiograph 4 years status post-PFA demonstrating degeneration of the lateral and medial compartments. The patient ultimately required conversion to TKA.

MODERN UKA OUTCOMES

Although early data were variable, more recent long-term series have demonstrated that with appropriate patient selection fixed-bearing UKA can render survivorship comparable with that of TKA. In the early 1990s, Scott and colleagues[36] reviewed results of 100 consecutive UKAs and reported a survivorship rate of 85% at 10 years and reported that 87% of patients were without significant pain. Romanowski and Repicci[37] reported good to excellent results in 86% of knees undergoing minimally invasive UKA at 8-year follow-up. Revision was performed in 10 patients because of advancement of disease in the remaining compartments (five patients); surgical error (three patients); poor pain relief (one patient); and periprosthetic fracture (one patient). In a report of patients with UKA younger than age 60, Swienckowski and colleagues[38] found that the 11-year survivorship was 92%. Berger and colleagues[39] used Kaplan-Meier analysis to demonstrate survival rates of 98% at 10-year and 95.7% at 13-year for 62 patients undergoing UKA. Additionally, at final follow-up there was no radiographic evidence of osteolysis or component loosening in any patient. With the same cohort, Foran and colleagues[40] reported 15-year and 20-year survivorship of 93% and 90%, respectively, again with no instances of loosening or osteolysis Likewise, in a series of 140 cemented UKAs, Squire and colleagues[41] reported a revision rate of 10% (comparable for fixed-bearing TKA) at average 18-year follow-up.

MOST COMMON MODES OF FAILURE

UKA can fail in several ways including polyethylene wear, adjacent tibiofemoral compartment and patellofemoral compartment degeneration, aseptic loosening, mechanical failure, malpositioned implants, and infection. Among these, polyethylene wear (with or without loosening) and progression of arthritis have been the most commonly reported modes of failure with modern UKA.[42–46] As demonstrated in the series by McAuley and colleagues[42] and Levine and colleagues,[43] these failure modes result in minimal bone loss and result in relatively straightforward revision procedures.

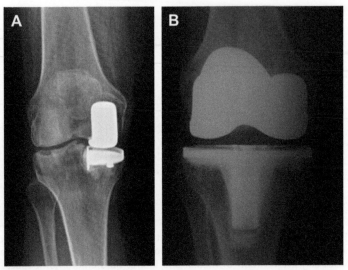

Fig. 5. (A) Patient with history of medial UKA with loose tibial component requiring revision. (B) Same patient postoperatively after conversion to TKA using primary TKA implants.

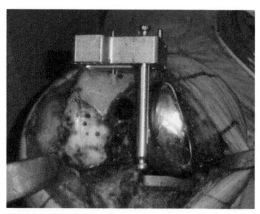

Fig. 6. Retention of the UKA femoral component can guide placement of the femoral cutting jig when converting from UKA to TKA.

McAuley and colleagues[42] revealed in a series of 39 UKA revisions that a primary femoral component could be used in all patients, and on the tibial side, the defects encountered were easily managed using autogenous nonstructural graft, wedges, and stems.

Popularity of UKA has also risen in light of ease of revision of UKA to TKA. Levine and colleagues[43] demonstrated that results of 31 UKA to TKA revisions at 45 months follow-up were superior to those of failed TKA and comparable with the authors' results of primary TKA at a similar follow-up interval. Springer and colleagues[47] converted 22 knees from UKA to TKA between 1993 and 2004 and noted good Knee Society score (93 ± standard deviation) and functional score (78 ± standard deviation) at an average of 64.5 months postoperatively. Johnson and colleagues[48] demonstrated a 10-year Kaplan-Meier survivorship of 91% in 77 knees converted from UKA to TKA. They concluded that revision of UKA to TKA is not technically difficult and provides results that are comparable with primary TKA (**Fig. 5**). Saldanha and colleagues[49] reported on 36 revision UKAs to TKA and demonstrated a mean total knee score of 86.3 and a mean functional score of 78.5 at average 2-year follow-up. They concluded that these results were better than revision TKA and they attributed these favorable results to preservation of bone stock and surrounding the soft tissue envelope. In our own experience, these revisions are facilitated by retention of the femoral component to use as a landmark for determining femoral component rotation and joint line restoration (**Fig. 6**).

SUMMARY

UKA has experienced resurgence in popularity because of the lower morbidity of the procedure and the proposed benefits over total knee replacement in appropriately selected patients. Improved component designs and advanced surgical techniques have promoted excellent results. In addition to the traditional criteria for UKA, expanded indications to include the very young and the elderly have yielded comparable clinical outcomes. Nonetheless, the success of unicompartmental replacement depends on proper surgical technique and patient selection. Distinct surgical considerations exist depending on whether the medial, lateral, or patellofemoral compartment is replaced. Although previously considered a staging procedure to postpone eventual need for total knee replacement, long-term studies have shown that unicompartmental knee replacement is an alternative to TKA.

REFERENCES

1. MacIntosh DL, Hunter GA. The use of the hemiarthroplasty prosthesis for advanced osteoarthritis and rheumatoid arthritis of the knee. J Bone Joint Surg Br 1972;54(2):244–55.
2. Emerson RH, Potter T. The use of the McKeever metallic hemiarthroplasty for unicompartmental arthritis. J Bone Joint Surg Am 1985;67(2):208–12.
3. Scott RD, Joyce MJ, Ewald FC, et al. McKeever metallic hemiarthroplasty of the knee in unicompartmental degenerative arthritis. Long-term clinical follow-up and current indications. J Bone Joint Surg Am 1985;67(2):203–7.
4. Springer BD, Scott RD, Sah AP, et al. McKeever hemiarthroplasty of the knee in patients less than sixty years old. J Bone Joint Surg Am 2006;88(2):366–71.
5. Insall J, Aglietti P. A five to seven-year follow-up of unicondylar arthroplasty. J Bone Joint Surg Am 1980;62(8):1329–37.
6. Laskin RS. Unicompartmental tibiofemoral resurfacing arthroplasty. J Bone Joint Surg Am 1978;60(2):182–5.
7. Thornhill TS. Unicompartmental knee arthroplasty. Clin Orthop Relat Res 1986;(205):121–31.
8. Capra SW, Fehring TK. Unicondylar arthroplasty. A survivorship analysis. J Arthroplasty 1992;7(3):247–51.
9. Kozinn SC, Marx C, Scott RD. Unicompartmental knee arthroplasty. A 4.5-6-year follow-up study with a metal-backed tibial component. J Arthroplasty 1989; 4(Suppl):S1–10.
10. Heck DA, Marmor L, Gibson A, et al. Unicompartmental knee arthroplasty. A multicenter investigation with long-term follow-up evaluation. Clin Orthop Relat Res 1993;(286):154–9.
11. Kozinn SC, Scott R. Unicondylar knee arthroplasty. J Bone Joint Surg Am 1989; 71(1):145–50.
12. Murray DW, Goodfellow JW, O'Connor JJ, et al. The Oxford medial unicompartmental arthroplasty: a ten-year survival study. J Bone Joint Surg Br 1998;80(6): 983–9.
13. Pandit H, Jenkins C, Gill HS, et al. Unnecessary contraindications for mobile-bearing unicompartmental knee replacement. J Bone Joint Surg Br 2011;93(5): 622–8.
14. Sah AP, Springer BD, Scott RD. Unicompartmental knee arthroplasty in octogenarians: survival longer than the patient. Clin Orthop Relat Res 2006;451: 107–12.
15. Goodfellow J, O'Connor J. The mechanics of the knee and prosthesis design. J Bone Joint Surg Br 1978;60(3):358–69.
16. Psychoyios V, Crawford RW, O'Connor JJ, et al. Wear of congruent meniscal bearings in unicompartmental knee arthroplasty: a retrieval study of 16 specimens. J Bone Joint Surg Br 1998;80(6):976–82.
17. Price AJ, Waite JC, Svard U. Long-term clinical results of the medial Oxford unicompartmental knee arthroplasty. Clin Orthop Relat Res 2005;(435):171–80.
18. Gunther TV, Murray DW, Miller R, et al. Lateral unicompartmental arthroplasty with the Oxford meniscal knee. In: The knee. 3rd edition; 1996. p. 33–9.
19. Repicci JA, Eberle RW. Minimally invasive surgical technique for unicondylar knee arthroplasty. J South Orthop Assoc 1999;8(1):20–7 [discussion: 27].

20. Fisher DA, Dalury DF, Adams MJ, et al. Unicompartmental and total knee arthroplasty in the over 70 population. Orthopedics 2010;33(9):668.
21. Brown NM, Sheth NP, Davis K, et al. Total knee arthroplasty has higher postoperative morbidity than unicompartmental knee arthroplasty: a multicenter analysis. J Arthroplasty 2012;27(Suppl 8):86–90.
22. Isaac SM, Barker KL, Danial IN, et al. Does arthroplasty type influence knee joint proprioception? A longitudinal prospective study comparing total and unicompartmental arthroplasty. Knee 2007;14(3):212–7.
23. Patil S, Colwell CW, Ezzet, KA, et al. Can normal knee kinematics be restored with unicompartmental knee replacement? J Bone Joint Surg Am 2005;87(2):332–8.
24. Scott RD. Lateral unicompartmental replacement: a road less traveled. Orthopedics 2005;28(9):983–4.
25. Sah AP, Scott RD. Lateral unicompartmental knee arthroplasty through a medial approach. Study with an average five-year follow-up. J Bone Joint Surg Am 2007; 89(9):1948–54.
26. Pennington DW, Swienckowski JJ, Lutes WB, et al. Lateral unicompartmental knee arthroplasty. J Arthroplasty 2006;21(1):13–7.
27. Walker T, Perkinson B, Mihalko WM. Patellofemoral arthroplasty: the other unicompartmental knee replacement. J Bone Joint Surg Am 2012;94(18):1712–20.
28. Krajca-Radcliffe JB, Coker TP. Patellofemoral arthroplasty. A 2- to 18-year followup study. Clin Orthop Relat Res 1996;(330):143–51.
29. Sisto DJ, Sarin VK. Custom patellofemoral arthroplasty of the knee. J Bone Joint Surg Am 2006;88(7):1475–80.
30. Dahm DL, Al-Rayashi W, Dajani K, et al. Patellofemoral arthroplasty versus total knee arthroplasty in patients with isolated patellofemoral osteoarthritis. Am J Orthop 2010;39(10):487–91.
31. Argenson JN, Flecher X, Parratte S, et al. Patellofemoral arthroplasty: an update. Clin Orthop Relat Res 2005;440:50–3.
32. Kooijman HJ, Driessen AP, van Horn JR. Long-term results of patellofemoral arthroplasty. A report of 56 arthroplasties with 17 years of follow-up. J Bone Joint Surg Br 2003;85(6):836–40.
33. Dalury DF, Fisher DA, Adams MJ, et al. Unicompartmental knee arthroplasty compares favorably to total knee arthroplasty in the same patient. Orthopedics 2009; 32(4).
34. Newman J, Pydisetty RV, Ackroyd C. Unicompartmental or total knee replacement: the 15-year results of a prospective randomised controlled trial. J Bone Joint Surg Br 2009;91(1):52–7.
35. Willis-Owen CA, Brust K, Alsop H, et al. Unicondylar knee arthroplasty in the UK National Health Service: an analysis of candidacy, outcome and cost efficacy. Knee 2009;16(6):473–8.
36. Scott RD, Cobb AG, McQueary FG, et al. Unicompartmental knee arthroplasty. Eight- to 12-year follow-up evaluation with survivorship analysis. Clin Orthop Relat Res 1991;(271):96–100.
37. Romanowski MR, Repicci JA. Minimally invasive unicondylar arthroplasty: eight-year follow-up. J Knee Surg 2002;15(1):17–22.
38. Swienckowski JJ, Pennington DW. Unicompartmental knee arthroplasty in patients sixty years of age or younger. J Bone Joint Surg Am 2004;86-A(Suppl 1(Pt 2)): 131–42.
39. Berger RA, Meneghini RM, Jacobs JJ, et al. Results of unicompartmental knee arthroplasty at a minimum of ten years of follow-up. J Bone Joint Surg Am 2005;87(5):999–1006.

40. Foran JR, Brown NM, Valle Della CJ, et al. Long-term survivorship and failure modes of unicompartmental knee arthroplasty. Clin Orthop Relat Res 2012; 471(1):102–8.

41. Squire MW, Callaghan JJ, Goetz DD, et al. Unicompartmental knee replacement. A minimum 15 year followup study. Clin Orthop Relat Res 1999;(367):61–72.

42. McAuley JP, Engh GA, Ammeen DJ. Revision of failed unicompartmental knee arthroplasty. Clin Orthop Relat Res 2001;(392):279–82.

43. Levine WN, Ozuna RM, Scott RD, et al. Conversion of failed modern unicompartmental arthroplasty to total knee arthroplasty. J Arthroplasty 1996;11(7):797–801.

44. Collier MB, Eickmann TH, Sukezaki F, et al. Patient, implant, and alignment factors associated with revision of medial compartment unicondylar arthroplasty. J Arthroplasty 2006;21(6):108–15.

45. Berger RA, Meneghini RM, Sheinkop MB, et al. The progression of patellofemoral arthrosis after medial unicompartmental replacement: results at 11 to 15 years. Clin Orthop Relat Res 2004;(428):92–9.

46. Aleto TJ, Berend ME, Ritter MA, et al. Early failure of unicompartmental knee arthroplasty leading to revision. Not Found In Database 2008;23(2):159–63.

47. Springer BD, Scott RD, Thornhill TS. Conversion of failed unicompartmental knee arthroplasty to TKA. Clin Orthop Relat Res 2006;446:214–20.

48. Johnson S, Jones P, Newman JH. The survivorship and results of total knee replacements converted from unicompartmental knee replacements. The Knee 2007;14(2):154–7.

49. Saldanha KA, Keys GW, Svard UC, et al. Revision of Oxford medial unicompartmental knee arthroplasty to total knee arthroplasty - results of a multicentre study. Knee 2007;14(4):275–9.

Future Trends for Unicompartmental Arthritis of the Knee: Injectables & Stem Cells

Marco Kawamura Demange, MD, PhD[a,b], Marco Sisto, BA[b],
Scott Rodeo, MD[b],*

KEYWORDS

- Arthritis • Knee arthritis • Injectable arthritis treatment • Osteoarthritis
- Hyaluronic acid • Stem cell

KEY POINTS

- Intra-articular corticosteroids and hyaluronic acid injections have a role in the treatment of early arthritis of the knee.
- Platelet-rich plasma (PRP) injections alone do not promote cartilage repair.
- The role of PRP injections in early knee osteoarthritis and focal cartilage lesions still needs to be better understood.
- Ultimately, combinations of various injectable materials may be useful in treating early knee osteoarthritis.
- Stem cell therapy has potential as either an isolated approach or combined with different surgical procedures.
- Gene therapy is a possibility but probably will not be available in the near future.

INTRODUCTION

Arthritis is one of the most frequent musculoskeletal problems, causing pain, disability, and a significant economic burden. In terms of prevalence, as life expectancy increases, arthritis prevalence will also increase.[1,2] There are estimates that osteoarthritis (OA) may become the fourth-highest impact condition in women and the eighth-most important condition in men in the developed world.[3]

There is no consensus about the best treatment option for early knee arthritis. Nonsurgical options include oral medications, injections, orthoses, physiotherapy, and lifestyle modification.[4,5] The main surgical options for arthritis of the knee after failure of a nonsurgical therapy include arthroscopic surgical procedures, cartilage repair

[a] Department of Orthopedic Surgery and Traumatology, University of São Paulo, Rua Ouvidio Pires de Campos, 333 São Paulo, SP 05403-010, Brazil; [b] Hospital for Special Surgery, Weil Cornell Medical College, 535 E 70th Street, New York, NY 10021, USA
* Corresponding author.
E-mail address: rodeos@hss.edu

Clin Sports Med 33 (2014) 161–174
http://dx.doi.org/10.1016/j.csm.2013.06.006
0278-5919/14/$ – see front matter © 2014 Elsevier Inc. All rights reserved.

or transplantation, realignment osteotomies, unicompartmental arthroplasties, or total knee arthroplasties.[4,5]

One of the main issues concerning early knee OA is that there are currently no treatment options that are able to completely revert the cartilage degenerative process. Ideally, the goal of nonsurgical treatments is to retard or stop the degenerative process. Despite the presence of unicompartmental arthritis, many patients still choose to participate in high-impact activities that can result in joint discomfort and pain. As a result, there has been a large effort to develop injectable treatments that relieve symptoms and delay the progression of early OA.

Cartilage focal lesions are also common in the adult population and may progress to arthritis.[6,7] Various knee disorders, including anterior cruciate ligament (ACL) tears,[8,9] meniscal tears and previous meniscectomies,[7] disruption of the subchondral bone,[10,11] and limb malalignment,[12] may lead to the development of cartilage lesions or progression to arthritis. Early treatment of focal cartilage lesions and early knee arthritis may be a possible approach to prevent progression of knee OA.[6,7,13–15]

In this article, we discuss current nonsurgical injectable treatment options, as well as future trends for cartilage lesions and early arthritis of the knee. We also cover some potential treatments for knee OA, including stem cell and gene therapies.[16,17]

CURRENT TREATMENT OPTIONS
Corticosteroid Injections

Corticosteroid injections have been performed in the treatment of knee OA for decades.[18,19] Recent systematic reviews have discussed the efficacy of corticosteroids compared with placebo. Similarly, recent studies have compared corticosteroids with other injectable treatment options, such as platelet-rich plasma (PRP) or hyaluronic acid (HA).[20] Corticosteroid injections may be performed alone, combined with other medications, or after knee arthroscopies.[16,21] The exact mechanism of the therapeutic effect of corticosteroids in knee OA is still unclear; however, it is believed to be related to the anti-inflammatory effect of the drug.[20] The short-term benefits of intra-articular corticosteroid injections are well established. The administration of steroid injections either alone or combined with local anesthetics has been shown to be a viable short-term option and is universally accepted in clinical practice as such.[22] The long-term benefits have not been confirmed and chronic use may lead to progressive cartilage degeneration. Maricar and colleagues[20] recently published a systematic review regarding intra-articular corticosteroid injection and predictors in knee OA. Within 696 publications, only 11 matched their inclusion criteria, but only 2 trials had a primary aim to determine predictors of response to corticosteroids. The investigators could not conclusively identify any predictors of response to intra-articular use of corticosteroids in knee OA, but they reported that synovitis and knee effusion may have some correlation with clinical improvement.[20]

Autologous-Conditioned Serum

Cytokines play an important role in the mechanism of OA. Interleukin-1 (IL-1) is known as one of the most important catabolic cytokines in the cartilage breakage process. The human body naturally produces an IL-1 receptor antagonist (IL-1ra), which is believed to have the potential to limit the intra-articular effects of the catabolic cytokine IL-1. Autologous-conditioned serum is generated by incubation of venous blood with glass beads.[23,24] After incubation for 24 hours at 37°C, the blood is recovered and centrifuged. Blood monocytes are a major natural source of IL-1ra and their production of IL-1ra is greatly stimulated by culture on immunoglobulin G–coated plates.

Woodell-May and colleagues[25] reported that the autologous protein solution (APS) contained both anabolic (basic fibroblast growth factor [bFGF], transforming growth factor [TGF]-β1, TGF-β2, epidermal growth factor [EGF], insulinlike growth factor [IGF]-1, platelet-derived growth factor [PDGF]-AB, PDGF-BB, and vascular endothelial growth factor [VEGF]) and anti-inflammatory (IL-1ra, sTNF-R1, sTNF-RII, IL-4, IL-10, IL- 13, and interferon-γ [IFNγ]) cytokines and that the combination of these cytokines is a potential candidate for treatment of OA. There are several animal studies evaluating the effect of autologous-conditioned serum; however, there are few clinical trials describing its efficacy. Baltzer and colleagues[26] performed a double-blinded randomized clinical trial comparing autologous conditioned serum (ACS) with hyaluronan and with saline. In this clinical trial, they enrolled 367 patients and found that ACS provided better pain relief and functional score (Western Ontario and McMaster Universities Osteoarthritis Index [WOMAC]) outcomes at 26 weeks of follow-up.

PRP Injections

PRP injections are considered a potential treatment option to improve joint function and decrease inflammatory mediator expression by delivering platelet-derived cytokines and growth factors to the affected area. IGF, especially IGF-1, is considered one of the main anabolic growth factors for articular cartilage.[27] IGF stimulates synthesis of integrins, type-II collagen, and proteoglycans; stimulates chondrocyte adhesion; improves tissue integration; and inhibits matrix degradation.[27,28] PDGF increases chondrocyte proliferation, but it seems to have more influence on meniscal cells than articular cartilage.[27,29] TGF-β1 is 1 of the 3 isoforms of TGF-β, and has its effects on chondrocytes and cartilage synthesis.[30] However, the mechanism of action of TGF-β1 is not completely understood, as it seems that there are significant differences between in vitro and in vivo behaviors. Also, in vivo TGF-β1 is released within the initial few days postinjury, compared with a long-lasting delivery of IGF-1. Some in vitro studies described that TGF-β1 may antagonize IGF-1 on glycosaminoglycan (GAG) synthesis when applied concomitantly.[30,31] PRP may modulate the function of human osteoarthritic chondrocytes by inhibiting the action of inflammatory cytokines, such as IL-1 and nuclear factor (NF)-kB.[32,33]

Clinical studies have demonstrated that PRP injections may decrease knee pain in patients with knee OA.[34] PRP may influence pain by inhibiting the action of inflammatory cytokines such as IL-1 and NF-kB. Patel and colleagues[34] compared leukocyte-free PRP and placebo injections in the treatment of patients with Ahlback grade 1 or 2 OA without significant deformity and observed improvement in pain scores at a minimum of 6-month follow-up with either single or double PRP injections. Spakova and colleagues[35] described better results with the use of PRP compared with HA injections at both 3-month and 6-month follow-up. Kon and colleagues[36,37] showed that pain scores improved with the use of PRP injections in arthritic joints. The results were stable from the end of the 3-injection cycle up to 6 months, but worsened at the 1-year[38] and 24-month[37] evaluations. The investigators described a trend for favorable results with PRP in patients with low-grade articular degeneration (Kellgren-Lawrence score up to 2).[39] On the other hand, a current systematic review performed by Sheth and colleagues[40] concluded that the evidence for the use of PRP knee injections is equivocal, as the literature still lacks evidence to support it. Halpern and colleagues[41] evaluated magnetic resonance images (MRIs) of the knee at baseline, 1 week, and 1, 3, 6, and 12 months after PRP injection in patients with OA. Pain scores significantly decreased, and functional and clinical scores increased at 6 months and 1 year from baseline. Qualitative MRIs demonstrated no change in at least 73% of cases at 1 year.

Hyaluronic Acid Injections

Knee arthritis may reduce the concentration of HA in the synovial fluid. HA is produced by type B synoviocytes and synovial fibroblasts. It is secreted into the joint where it acts as a lubricant, shock absorber, extracellular matrix scaffold, and chondroprotective milieu facilitating chondrocyte nutrition.[42] Viscosupplementation involves intra-articular injection of a viscoelastic mucopolysaccharide component of synovial fluid (HA) after aspiration of any existing joint effusion.[43] HA is a high-molecular-weight glycosaminoglycan that consists of a repeating sequence of disaccharide units composed of N-acetyl glucosamine and glucuronic acid.[42,43] Initially, the idea of HA injection was to reestablish the normal synovial fluid viscoelastic properties. This initial hypothesis of how HA injection would act in OA joints has not been fully proven at this time, and we still do not understand the mechanism of action of HA injections.[32,44,45]

There is still some controversy about the clinical efficacy of HA viscosupplementation in the treatment of knee OA.[46] Rutjes and colleagues[47] recently published a systematic review analyzing articles from the MEDLINE (1996–2012), EMBASE (1980–2012), and Cochrane Center Register of Controlled Trials (1970–2012) databases. Their data included 89 trials involving 12,667 adults. The investigators described that 71 trials (9617 patients) showed that viscosupplementation moderately reduced pain and 18 trials showed a clinically irrelevant effect size.

FUTURE TRENDS

There is a great effort toward developing less-invasive and more "regenerative" approaches in the treatment of cartilage lesions and OA. For advanced arthritis, it seems to be more difficult to reverse the established cartilage degeneration. In the case of focal cartilage lesions and early arthritis, new approaches may be able to repair or even regenerate functional tissue, as well as slow the progression of OA. Even though we are focusing our discussion on injectables and stem cells in this article, we certainly need to emphasize that combining surgical correction of predisposing factors, such as mechanical malalignment, knee instability, or meniscus deficiency, is probably equal or more important to the treatments discussed here.

Corticosteroids

There has been very little research into creating new or modifying current corticosteroid intra-articular injections. Developing a sustained delivery of the drug into the joint is one research area. Combining corticosteroid injections with other therapies may also be another trend to its future use. Kinase inhibitors, such as p38 inhibitors, may help to improve corticosteroid effects.[48,49] To our knowledge, there is one private company performing preclinical, phase1, and phase 2 trials with new products for knee OA involving p38 inhibition, sustained effect corticosteroids, and tyrosine kinase A (TrkA) inhibitors.[50]

Lubricants and Viscosupplementation

HA formulations currently available for clinical use are quite varied, differing in molecular weight, method of production, and possibly half-life in the joint.[42] To increase the HA half-life in the joint, different cross-linking procedures are being researched. Cross-linking is a process in which the individual chains of HA are chemically bound (or "cross-linked") together, creating a more viscous substance, transforming it from a liquid into a "gel." The firmness of the gel depends on the degree of cross-linking.[51] The body metabolizes cross-linked HA slower than the non–cross linked, which may result in a longer-lasting effect in the knee joint.

Developments in the research of HA cross-linkage have resulted in highly visco-elastic materials that may be capable of preparation in a mixture of relevant growth hormones or anti-inflammatory drugs.[52,53]

New synthetic lubricants that mimic natural joint synovial fluid substances are also being studied. Lubricin (also known as superficial zone protein) is one of the primary lubricating substances in diarthrodial joints, being responsible for the lubrication of pressurized cartilage. It is mucinous glycoprotein produced by synovial fibroblasts and superficial zone articular chondrocytes. Lubricin expression is downregulated by proinflammatory cytokines, such as IL-1 and tumor necrosis factor (TNF)-alpha and upregulated by TGF-β and bone morphogenic protein (BMP)-7.[54,55] Some OA animal-model studies have demonstrated that synthetic lubricin provides a chondro-protective effect,[56] which may be more effective than HA injections.[57]

Growth Factor–Related Injections

A greater understanding of the cytokine cascades associated with OA and OA pro-gression may lead to the development of new biologic injections. Current knowledge supports that IL-1 beta is the main cytokine in the degenerative arthritis process, and research on IL-1ra is a promising area. Substances such as IGF-1,[27,58] TGF-β, FGF-18,[59] as well as anti-inflammatory cytokines such as IL-4 and IL-10,[60] PDGF,[27] and adrenomedullin,[61] may play a role in the development of new therapies. IGF-1 is a pro-anabolic cytokine to chondrocytes, stimulating matrix deposition and, to a lesser extent, cell proliferation.

Most studies are in the preclinical phase, consisting mainly of small animal research, which may lead to clinical studies in the near future. For example, Van Meegeren and colleagues[60] demonstrated in a mouse model that a single intra-articular injection of IL-4 plus IL-10 directly after a single joint bleed limits cartilage degeneration over time. Yorimitsu and colleagues[62] demonstrated that IL-4 might promote a chondro-protective response to mechanical stress-induced cartilage destruction in OA rat models. Although some of the potential benefits of cytokine or cytokine-antagonist injections have been shown in animal studies, clinical studies concerning long-term safety of biotherapy injections is mandatory, as exposing patients to serious side effects is not acceptable in a benign disease such as OA.[63]

Inhibition of the degradative effects of matrix metalloproteinases (MMPs) to prevent cartilage and joint destruction may become another future treatment option for early OA. The family of proteolytic enzymes responsible for OA cartilage matrix digestion is the MMPs.[64] Collagenases, particularly collagenase-1 (MMP-1) and collagenase-3 (MMP-13), are involved in type II collagen degradation. Stromelysin-1 (MMP-3) and aggrecanase-1 (ADAMTS-4) have been shown to play a primary role in the degra-dation of proteoglycans.[65] Most studies on MMP inhibitors are related to rheumatoid arthritis,[66] but their mechanism of action might help degenerative arthritis treatment as well.[67] Doxycycline has been shown to inhibit MMP activity, and is currently being investigated as a disease-modifying agent in OA, but is still not recommended for clin-ical use.[68]

Stem Cells

Stem cells are capable of long-term proliferation, self-renewal, and differentiation into many cell types and lineages. Because of their proliferative potential, stem cells are implicated as being capable of providing tissue repair and regeneration. Stem cells may be classified as embryonic or nonembryonic (somatic or adult) stem cells.

Embryonic stem cells are derived from embryos and have the potential to proliferate without differentiating. The regulatory and governmental restrictions regarding embryonic stem cells limit research, as well as the further involvement of these cells for intra-articular injections. Induced pluripotent stem cells (iPSCs) are derived from a nonpluripotent cell (adult somatic cell) by "reprogramming" the cells by transfection with specific genes.[69] The iPSCs have similar functional capability as embryonic stem cells and, as they are developed from a patient's own somatic cells, they may not lead to a significant immunogenic response.[69]

Adult stem cells are undifferentiated cells found among differentiated cells in a tissue or organ; these represent a progenitor cell population with multipotent potential.[70] Adult stem cells do not have the plasticity of embryonic stem cells, but they may differentiate into multiple lineages of their tissue of origin or undergo significantly more replicative cycles than other cells. Adult stem cells found in the bone marrow are classified either as hematopoietic stem cells and bone marrow stromal stem cells (or mesenchymal stem cells [MSCs]).[70] The hematopoietic stem cells form all types of blood cells, whereas the adult MSCs differentiate into different mesenchymal tissues, which include bone, tendon, cartilage, fat, or muscle. Neural stem cells, epithelial stem cells, and hematopoietic stem cells are not currently a focus for musculoskeletal applications, as MSCs are the main cell type being investigated for treatment of OA.[70,71]

One of the main questions in the use of stem cells is how to identify exactly how cells differentiate and to identify the fate of these cells in the target tissue. Under appropriate culture conditions, MSCs are capable of differentiating into the osteogenic, chondrogenic, myogenic, and adipogenic lineages.[72,73]

Safety issues are usually discussed regarding stem cell therapy. Centeno and colleagues[74] recently published a 339 patient surveillance study with no neoplastic complications. In this study, the average follow-up was 11.3 months and the maximum follow-up was 4 years. Wakitani and colleagues[75] reported that 41 patients received MSC autologous implantations with no carcinogenic or infection complications after an average follow-up of 75 months (range 5–137 months).

Stem cells may be used clinically in cell suspension, as concentrates, or expanded by culture.[73,76] They can be delivered through knee injections or combined with surgical procedures.[73] Several MSC cell sources have being evaluated for cartilage repair, including cells derived from bone marrow,[77] periosteoum,[77] synovial tissue,[78,79] adipose tissue[80] and infrapatellar fat-pad.[81] Emadedin and colleagues[82] described a case series of 6 female patients who had received intra-articular injection of MSCs. The MSC samples were obtained by bone marrow aspiration and isolated in the laboratory. The investigators described increases in cartilage thickness as well as decreases in subchondral bone edema. Centeno and colleagues[83] reported cartilage growth in one patient following cultured bone-derived MSC injection. Pak[84] reported 2 patients older than 70 years with knee OA treated with MSC injections resulting in a reduction of knee pain.

Synovial-derived stem cells are described as the tissue-specific cells for cartilage regeneration.[79,85] Koh and colleagues[86] described a case series of 18 patients who received intra-articular injections of adipose synovium-derived autologous mesenchymal stem cells for treatment of OA. The investigators described that the injections reduced knee pain, improved knee function, and improved cartilage score on MRI evaluation. Davatchi and colleagues[87] reported 4 patients with moderate to severe OA treated with cultured bone marrow–derived MSCs (BMMSCs) that demonstrated clinical improvement at 6-month follow-up.

Umbilical cord cells and fetal stem cells would seem to have tremendous potential for cartilage repair.[88,89] However, to date there is very little information available. These cell sources may be viable option from a biologic perspective, but clinical use will require further research, consideration of ethical issues, and changes in the regulatory environment.

The resultant cartilage degeneration after partial meniscectomy has led to clinical trials examining the safety and efficacy of single intra-articular stem cell injections. These injections can vary widely and usually differ in human MSC (hMSC) concentration and injection vehicle make-up. Ongoing OA studies to determine the most effective use of hMSCs have used methods of cell delivery such as suspension in commercial sodium hyaluronan or diluted hyaluronan.[90]

Currently there is lack of clinical reports on stem cell injections in the knee. Most studies have evaluated cells used at the time of cartilage repair surgical procedures. MSCs have been evaluated for treatment of focal articular cartilage defects using 1-step MSC isolation from bone marrow concentrates or using cultured MSCs.[75] MSC implantation technique and cartilage lesion debridement is similar to autologous chondrocyte implantation surgery in the treatment of focal chondral lesions.[75,91,92] Buda and colleagues[91] described technical aspects of the surgical treatment of osteochondral lesions in the knee with MSC as a single-step procedure.[91] This procedure involves aspirating bone marrow before the surgical procedure, separating BMMSCs by centrifugation, and injecting them into the cartilage defect using a scaffold.[91] In 2004, Wakitani and colleagues[93] reported 2 patients treated with cultured BMMSCs for full-thickness patella cartilage lesions. Nejadnik and colleagues[94] reported their results comparing a cohort of 36 patients treated with autologous chondrocyte implantation (ACI) and a cohort of 36 patients treated with cultured BMMSC. The investigators reported no statistically significant difference between the 2 treatments in functional evaluation. The investigators also obtained biopsies of 7 patients (4 in the BMMSC group and 3 in ACI group) during second-look arthroscopy demonstrating hyalinelike cartilage in both. Potentially, these approaches may even be used to treat early unicompartmental arthritis with normal subchondral bone.[95,96]

Gene Therapy

Gene therapy is the process of genetically modifying cells to alter the expression of one or more genes in an effort to exert a therapeutic effect. Gene therapy can be administered directly to an organism (in vivo) or to explanted cells or tissues that can then be reimplanted or injected (ex vivo).[45,97] A vector carrying the gene of interest is loaded into the cell. This process inserts the new genetic material (DNA) into the cell to induce expression of the desired transgenes.[45] Theoretically, gene therapy in the knee offers the benefit of the exposure being restricted to the local intra-articular space, which not only avoids systemic side effects but also should provide a longer-lasting effect.[45] The synovial cells are possibly the easiest target cells for intra-articular transgene expression, as they are largely available and accessible inside the knee.

Clinical use of gene therapy in the knee seems to be a more distant reality because of the several clinical safety trials that are needed before widespread clinical use. Ha and colleagues[98] have performed a phase I safety study of retroviral transduced human chondrocytes expressing transforming growth factor-beta-1 in degenerative arthritis patients, and they reported no safety issues. Animal model studies have illustrated both the potential positive and potential negative effects of gene therapy. Hsieh and colleagues[99] demonstrated that thrombospodin-1 might suppress OA progression in a rat model experiment.[90] On the other hand, Watson and colleagues[100] demonstrated knee arthrofibrosis after adenovirus injection to overexpress TGF-β1 in rat knee joints. Additional intracellular and extracellular growth and differentiation regulators that may serve as suitable constituents include parathyroid hormone–related protein,[101] Indian Hedgehog,[64,102] retinoic acid,[103–105] wnt-β-catenin,[106,107] SOX9,[108–111] CART-1,[112,113] and runt.[114]

Gene therapy may be the most promising treatment for long-term cytokine delivery into the knee.[45] However, further study is required, and gene therapy techniques are not expected to be clinically available in the short term.

FINAL CONSIDERATIONS

Our protocol is to start with a corticosteroid injection if there are any signs of active synovitis or effusion. If the symptoms are rather just chronic, activity-related pain with no evidence of an effusion, we may consider HA injection as the first-line treatment, because of the potential for HA to provide longer duration of relief. On occasion, combined injection of a corticosteroid and HA may be considered, and appears to be safe. PRP or autologous conditioned serum is uncommonly used in our current treatment protocol, based on the variability in different preparations, modest reported efficacy, and cost. We do not currently recommend injections in a prophylactic manner, given the lack of any evidence that any injectable substance can affect the structure and/or composition of articular cartilage. Perhaps in the future, substances such as lubricin-mimetics or substances that affect production of proinflammatory mediators, MMPs, or other catabolic factors may have a role in prevention of posttraumatic arthrosis. Stem cell injections are not currently used in our practice for nonoperative treatment of the injured joint. Stem cell approaches will be a more viable approach in the United States once the Food and Drug Administration guidelines allow culturing and manipulation of autologous cell aspirates.

In the future, knee injections may be used as a nonsurgical approach, as well as associated with surgical procedures. Currently most approaches are symptom-modifying, based on providing pain relief and improvement of symptoms, but certainly future approaches will aim to be structure-modifying or even regenerative treatments.

REFERENCES

1. Leyland KM, Hart DJ, Javaid MK, et al. The natural history of radiographic knee osteoarthritis: a fourteen-year population-based cohort study. Arthritis Rheum 2012;64:2243–51.
2. Felson DT, Zhang Y, Hannan MT, et al. The incidence and natural history of knee osteoarthritis in the elderly. The Framingham Osteoarthritis Study. Arthritis Rheum 1995;38:1500–5.
3. Murray CJ, Lopesz AD. The global burden of disease: a comprehensive assessment of mortality and disability from diseases, injuries, and risk factors in 1990 and projected to 2020. Cambridge (United Kingdom): Harvard School of Public Health, on behalf of the World Health Organization; 1996.
4. McAlindon T, Zucker NV, Zucker MO. 2007 OARSI recommendations for the management of hip and knee osteoarthritis: towards consensus? Osteoarthr Cartil 2008;16:636–7.
5. Zhang W, Moskowitz RW, Nuki G, et al. OARSI recommendations for the management of hip and knee osteoarthritis, part I: critical appraisal of existing treatment guidelines and systematic review of current research evidence. Osteoarthr Cartil 2007;15:981–1000.
6. Davies-Tuck ML, Wluka AE, Wang Y, et al. The natural history of cartilage defects in people with knee osteoarthritis. Osteoarthr Cartil 2008;16:337–42.
7. Widuchowski W, Widuchowski J, Trzaska T. Articular cartilage defects: study of 25,124 knee arthroscopies. Knee 2007;14:177–82.

8. Neuman P, Englund M, Kostogiannis I, et al. Prevalence of tibiofemoral osteoarthritis 15 years after nonoperative treatment of anterior cruciate ligament injury: a prospective cohort study. Am J Sports Med 2008;36:1717–25.
9. Amin S, Guermazi A, Lavalley MP, et al. Complete anterior cruciate ligament tear and the risk for cartilage loss and progression of symptoms in men and women with knee osteoarthritis. Osteoarthr Cartil 2008;16:897–902.
10. Guymer E, Baranyay F, Wluka AE, et al. A study of the prevalence and associations of subchondral bone marrow lesions in the knees of healthy, middle-aged women. Osteoarthr Cartil 2007;15:1437–42.
11. Davies-Tuck ML, Wluka AE, Wang Y, et al. The natural history of bone marrow lesions in community-based adults with no clinical knee osteoarthritis. Ann Rheum Dis 2009;68:904–8.
12. Felson DT, Goggins J, Niu J, et al. The effect of body weight on progression of knee osteoarthritis is dependent on alignment. Arthritis Rheum 2004;50:3904–9.
13. Wang Y, Ding C, Wluka AE, et al. Factors affecting progression of knee cartilage defects in normal subjects over 2 years. Rheumatology (Oxford) 2006;45:79–84.
14. Cameron M, Buchgraber A, Passler H, et al. The natural history of the anterior cruciate ligament-deficient knee. Changes in synovial fluid cytokine and keratan sulfate concentrations. Am J Sports Med 1997;25:751–4.
15. Chang A, Hochberg M, Song J, et al. Frequency of varus and valgus thrust and factors associated with thrust presence in persons with or at higher risk of developing knee osteoarthritis. Arthritis Rheum 2010;62:1403–11.
16. van Oosterhout M, Sont JK, Bajema IM, et al. Comparison of efficacy of arthroscopic lavage plus administration of corticosteroids, arthroscopic lavage plus administration of placebo, and joint aspiration plus administration of corticosteroids in arthritis of the knee: a randomized controlled trial. Arthritis Rheum 2006;55:964–70.
17. Ding C, Jones G, Wluka AE, et al. What can we learn about osteoarthritis by studying a healthy person against a person with early onset of disease? Curr Opin Rheumatol 2010;22:520–7.
18. Hollander JL. The local effects of compound F (hydrocortisone) injected into joints. Bull Rheum Dis 1951;2:3–4.
19. Schumacher HR, Chen LX. Injectable corticosteroids in treatment of arthritis of the knee. Am J Med 2005;118:1208 14.
20. Maricar N, Callaghan MJ, Felson DT, et al. Predictors of response to intra-articular steroid injections in knee osteoarthritis—a systematic review. Rheumatology (Oxford) 2012;52(6):1022–32.
21. Smith MD, Wetherall M, Darby T, et al. A randomized placebo-controlled trial of arthroscopic lavage versus lavage plus intra-articular corticosteroids in the management of symptomatic osteoarthritis of the knee. Rheumatology (Oxford) 2003;42:1477–85.
22. Hepper CT, Halvorson JJ, Duncan ST, et al. The efficacy and duration of intra-articular corticosteroid injection for knee osteoarthritis: a systematic review of level I studies. J Am Acad Orthop Surg 2009;17:638–46.
23. Wehling P, Moser C, Frisbie D, et al. Autologous conditioned serum in the treatment of orthopedic diseases: the orthokine therapy. BioDrugs 2007;21:323–32.
24. Meijer H, Reinecke J, Becker C, et al. The production of anti-inflammatory cytokines in whole blood by physico-chemical induction. Inflamm Res 2003;52:404–7.
25. Woodell-May J, Matuska A, Oyster M, et al. Autologous protein solution inhibits MMP-13 production by IL-1beta and TNFalpha-stimulated human articular chondrocytes. J Orthop Res 2011;29:1320–6.

26. Baltzer AW, Moser C, Jansen SA, et al. Autologous conditioned serum (Orthokine) is an effective treatment for knee osteoarthritis. Osteoarthr Cartil 2009;17:152–60.

27. Schmidt MB, Chen EH, Lynch SE. A review of the effects of insulin-like growth factor and platelet derived growth factor on in vivo cartilage healing and repair. Osteoarthr Cartil 2006;14:403–12.

28. Tumia NS, Johnstone AJ. Regional regenerative potential of meniscal cartilage exposed to recombinant insulin-like growth factor-I in vitro. J Bone Joint Surg Br 2004;86:1077–81.

29. Tumia NS, Johnstone AJ. Platelet derived growth factor-AB enhances knee meniscal cell activity in vitro. The Knee 2009;16:73–6.

30. Patil AS, Sable RB, Kothari RM. An update on transforming growth factor-beta (TGF-beta): sources, types, functions and clinical applicability for cartilage/bone healing. J Cell Physiol 2011;226:3094–103.

31. Delatte ML, Von den Hoff JW, Nottet SJ, et al. Growth regulation of the rat mandibular condyle and femoral head by transforming growth factor-{beta}1, fibroblast growth factor-2 and insulin-like growth factor-I. Eur J Orthod 2005; 27:17–26.

32. Dinarello CA. The role of the interleukin-1-receptor antagonist in blocking inflammation mediated by interleukin-1. N Engl J Med 2000;343:732–4.

33. van Buul GM, Koevoet WL, Kops N, et al. Platelet-rich plasma releasate inhibits inflammatory processes in osteoarthritic chondrocytes. Am J Sports Med 2011; 39:2362–70.

34. Patel S, Dhillon MS, Aggarwal S, et al. Treatment with platelet-rich plasma is more effective than placebo for knee osteoarthritis: a prospective, double-blind, randomized trial. Am J Sports Med 2013;41(2):356–64.

35. Spakova T, Rosocha J, Lacko M, et al. Treatment of knee joint osteoarthritis with autologous platelet-rich plasma in comparison with hyaluronic acid. Am J Phys Med Rehabil 2012;91(5):411–7.

36. Kon E, Mandelbaum B, Buda R, et al. Platelet-rich plasma intra-articular injection versus hyaluronic acid viscosupplementation as treatments for cartilage pathology: from early degeneration to osteoarthritis. Arthroscopy 2011;27:1490–501.

37. Filardo G, Kon E, Buda R, et al. Platelet-rich plasma intra-articular knee injections for the treatment of degenerative cartilage lesions and osteoarthritis. Knee Surg Sports Traumatol Arthrosc 2011;19:528–35.

38. Kon E, Buda R, Filardo G, et al. Platelet-rich plasma: intra-articular knee injections produced favorable results on degenerative cartilage lesions. Knee Surg Sports Traumatol Arthrosc 2010;18:472–9.

39. Filardo G, Kon E, Di Martino A, et al. Platelet-rich plasma vs hyaluronic acid to treat knee degenerative pathology: study design and preliminary results of a randomized controlled trial. BMC Musculoskelet Disord 2012;13:229.

40. Sheth U, Simunovic N, Klein G, et al. Efficacy of autologous platelet-rich plasma use for orthopaedic indications: a meta-analysis. J Bone Joint Surg Am 2012;94: 298–307.

41. Halpern B, Chaudhury S, Rodeo SA, et al. Clinical and MRI outcomes after platelet-rich plasma treatment for knee osteoarthritis. Clin J Sport Med 2013; 23(3):238–9.

42. Strauss EJ, Hart JA, Miller MD, et al. Hyaluronic acid viscosupplementation and osteoarthritis: current uses and future directions. Am J Sports Med 2009;37: 1636–44.

43. Brockmeier SF, Shaffer BS. Viscosupplementation therapy for osteoarthritis. Sports Med Arthrosc 2006;14:155–62.

44. Dunn S, Kolomytkin OV, Marino AA. Pathophysiology of osteoarthritis: evidence against the viscoelastic theory. Pathobiology 2009;76:322–8.
45. Evans CH. Novel biological approaches to the intra-articular treatment of osteoarthritis. BioDrugs 2005;19:355–62.
46. Zhang W, Nuki G, Moskowitz RW, et al. OARSI recommendations for the management of hip and knee osteoarthritis: part III: changes in evidence following systematic cumulative update of research published through 2009. Osteoarthr Cartil 2010;18:476–99.
47. Rutjes AW, Juni P, da Costa BR, et al. Viscosupplementation for osteoarthritis of the knee: a systematic review and meta-analysis. Ann Intern Med 2012;157:180–91.
48. Kyttaris VC. Kinase inhibitors: a new class of antirheumatic drugs. Drug Des Devel Ther 2012;6:245–50.
49. Balague C, Pont M, Prats N, et al. Profiling of dihydroorotate dehydrogenase, p38 and JAK inhibitors in the rat adjuvant-induced arthritis model: a translational study. Br J Pharmacol 2012;166:1320–32.
50. Flexion Therapeutics 2013, FX006 in the treatment of inflammation, Available at: http://www.flexiontherapeutics.com/programs/.
51. Segura T, Anderson BC, Chung PH, et al. Crosslinked hyaluronic acid hydrogels: a strategy to functionalize and pattern. Biomaterials 2005;26:359–71.
52. Palmieri B, Rottigni V, Iannitti T. Preliminary study of highly cross-linked hyaluronic acid-based combination therapy for management of knee osteoarthritis-related pain. Drug Des Devel Ther 2013;7:7–12.
53. Strand V, Baraf HS, Lavin PT, et al. A multicenter, randomized controlled trial comparing a single intra-articular injection of Gel-200, a new cross-linked formulation of hyaluronic acid, to phosphate buffered saline for treatment of osteoarthritis of the knee. Osteoarthr Cartil 2012;20:350–6.
54. Jones AR, Flannery CR. Bioregulation of lubricin expression by growth factors and cytokines. Eur Cell Mater 2007;13:40–5 [discussion: 5].
55. Yamane S, Reddi AH. Induction of chondrogenesis and superficial zone protein accumulation in synovial side population cells by BMP-7 and TGF-beta1. J Orthop Res 2008;26:485–92.
56. Jay GD, Fleming BC, Watkins BA, et al. Prevention of cartilage degeneration and restoration of chondroprotection by lubricin tribosupplementation in the rat following anterior cruciate ligament transection. Arthritis Rheum 2010;62:2382–91.
57. Teeple E, Elsaid KA, Jay GD, et al. Effects of supplemental intra-articular lubricin and hyaluronic acid on the progression of posttraumatic arthritis in the anterior cruciate ligament-deficient rat knee. Am J Sports Med 2011;39:164–72.
58. Sakimura K, Matsumoto T, Miyamoto C, et al. Effects of insulin-like growth factor I on transforming growth factor beta1 induced chondrogenesis of synovium-derived mesenchymal stem cells cultured in a polyglycolic acid scaffold. Cells Tissues Organs 2006;183:55–61.
59. Moore EE, Bendele AM, Thompson DL, et al. Fibroblast growth factor-18 stimulates chondrogenesis and cartilage repair in a rat model of injury-induced osteoarthritis. Osteoarthr Cartil 2005;13:623–31.
60. van Meegeren ME, Roosendaal G, Coeleveld K, et al. A single intra-articular injection with IL-4 plus IL-10 ameliorates blood-induced cartilage degeneration in haemophilic mice. Br J Haematol 2013;160(4):515–20.
61. Okura T, Marutsuka K, Hamada H, et al. Therapeutic efficacy of intra-articular adrenomedullin injection in antigen-induced arthritis in rabbits. Arthritis Res Ther 2008;10:R133.

62. Yorimitsu M, Nishida K, Shimizu A, et al. Intra-articular injection of interleukin-4 decreases nitric oxide production by chondrocytes and ameliorates subsequent destruction of cartilage in instability-induced osteoarthritis in rat knee joints. Osteoarthr Cartil 2008;16:764–71.

63. Chevalier X, Conrozier T, Richette P. Desperately looking for the right target in osteoarthritis: the anti-IL-1 strategy. Arthritis Res Ther 2011;13:124.

64. Wei F, Zhou J, Wei X, et al. Activation of Indian hedgehog promotes chondrocyte hypertrophy and upregulation of MMP-13 in human osteoarthritic cartilage. Osteoarthr Cartil 2012;20:755–63.

65. Munhoz FB, Godoy-Santos AL, Santos MC. MMP-3 polymorphism: genetic marker in pathological processes (Review). Mol Med Rep 2010;3:735–40.

66. Oliver SJ, Firestein GS, Arsenault L, et al. Vanadate, an inhibitor of stromelysin and collagenase expression, suppresses collagen induced arthritis. J Rheumatol 2007;34:1802–9.

67. Nasu Y, Nishida K, Miyazawa S, et al. A histone deacetylase inhibitor, suppresses synovial inflammation and subsequent cartilage destruction in a collagen antibody-induced arthritis mouse model. Osteoarthr Cartil 2008;16:723–32.

68. da Costa BR, Nuesch E, Reichenbach S, et al. Doxycycline for osteoarthritis of the knee or hip. Cochrane Database Syst Rev 2012;(11):CD007323.

69. Diekman BO, Christoforou N, Willard VP, et al. Cartilage tissue engineering using differentiated and purified induced pluripotent stem cells. Proc Natl Acad Sci U S A 2012;109:19172–7.

70. Caplan AI. Adult mesenchymal stem cells for tissue engineering versus regenerative medicine. J Cell Physiol 2007;213:341–7.

71. Koga H, Engebretsen L, Brinchmann JE, et al. Mesenchymal stem cell-based therapy for cartilage repair: a review. Knee Surg Sports Traumatol Arthrosc 2009;17:1289–97.

72. Barry FP. Mesenchymal stem cell therapy in joint disease. Novartis Found Symp 2003;249:86–96 [discussion: 96–102, 170–4, 239–41].

73. Krampera M, Pizzolo G, Aprili G, et al. Mesenchymal stem cells for bone, cartilage, tendon and skeletal muscle repair. Bone 2006;39:678–83.

74. Centeno CJ, Schultz JR, Cheever M, et al. Safety and complications reporting update on the re-implantation of culture-expanded mesenchymal stem cells using autologous platelet lysate technique. Curr Stem Cell Res Ther 2011;6: 368–78.

75. Wakitani S, Okabe T, Horibe S, et al. Safety of autologous bone marrow-derived mesenchymal stem cell transplant for cartilage repair in 41 patients with 45 joints followed for up to 11 years and 5 months. J Tissue Eng Regen Med 2011;5:146–50.

76. Filardo G, Madry H, Jelic M, et al. Mesenchymal stem cells for the treatment of cartilage lesions: from preclinical findings to clinical application in orthopaedics. Knee Surg Sports Traumatol Arthrosc 2013. [Epub ahead of print].

77. Wakitani S, Goto T, Pineda SJ, et al. Mesenchymal cell-based repair of large, full-thickness defects of articular cartilage. J Bone Joint Surg Am 1994;76:579–92.

78. Pei M, He F, Vunjak-Novakovic G. Synovium-derived stem cell-based chondrogenesis. Differentiation 2008;76:1044–56.

79. Pei M, He F, Li J, et al. Repair of large animal partial-thickness cartilage defects through intraarticular injection of matrix-rejuvenated synovium-derived stem cells. Tissue Eng Part A 2013;19(9–10):1144–54.

80. Guilak F, Estes BT, Diekman BO, et al. 2010 Nicolas Andry Award: multipotent adult stem cells from adipose tissue for musculoskeletal tissue engineering. Clin Orthop Relat Res 2010;468:2530–40.

81. Wickham MQ, Erickson GR, Gimble JM, et al. Multipotent stromal cells derived from the infrapatellar fat pad of the knee. Clin Orthop Relat Res 2003;(412): 196–212.
82. Emadedin M, Aghdami N, Taghiyar L, et al. Intra-articular injection of autologous mesenchymal stem cells in six patients with knee osteoarthritis. Arch Iran Med 2012;15:422–8.
83. Centeno CJ, Busse D, Kisiday J, et al. Increased knee cartilage volume in degenerative joint disease using percutaneously implanted, autologous mesenchymal stem cells. Pain Physician 2008;11:343–53.
84. Pak J. Regeneration of human bones in hip osteonecrosis and human cartilage in knee osteoarthritis with autologous adipose-tissue-derived stem cells: a case series. J Med Case Rep 2011;5:296.
85. Sakaguchi Y, Sekiya I, Yagishita K, et al. Comparison of human stem cells derived from various mesenchymal tissues: superiority of synovium as a cell source. Arthritis Rheum 2005;52:2521–9.
86. Koh YG, Jo SB, Kwon OR, et al. Mesenchymal stem cell injections improve symptoms of knee osteoarthritis. Arthroscopy 2013;29(4):748–55.
87. Davatchi F, Abdollahi BS, Mohyeddin M, et al. Mesenchymal stem cell therapy for knee osteoarthritis. Preliminary report of four patients. Int J Rheum Dis 2011; 14:211–5.
88. van Gool SA, Emons JA, Leijten JC, et al. Fetal mesenchymal stromal cells differentiating towards chondrocytes acquire a gene expression profile resembling human growth plate cartilage. PLoS One 2012;7:e44561.
89. Arufe MC, De la Fuente A, Fuentes I, et al. Umbilical cord as a mesenchymal stem cell source for treating joint pathologies. World J Orthopedics 2011;2: 43–50.
90. McCulloch S, Follow-up study of chondrogen delivered by intra-articular injection following meniscectomy. 2010 (Accessed Identifier: NCT00702741). Registered clinical trial available at: http://www.clinicaltrials.gov/ct2/show/record/NCT00702741?term5Chondrogen&rank51.
91. Buda R, Vannini F, Cavallo M, et al. Osteochondral lesions of the knee: a new one-step repair technique with bone-marrow-derived cells. J Bone Joint Surg Am 2010;92(Suppl 2):2–11.
92. Matsumoto T, Okabe T, Ikawa T, et al. Articular cartilage repair with autologous bone marrow mesenchymal cells. J Cell Physiol 2010;225:291–5.
93. Wakitani S, Mitsuoka T, Nakamura N, et al. Autologous bone marrow stromal cell transplant for repair of full-thickness articular cartilage defects in human patellae: two case reports. Cell Transplant 2004;13:595–600.
94. Nejadnik H, Hui JH, Feng Choong EP, et al. Autologous bone marrow-derived mesenchymal stem cells versus autologous chondrocyte implantation: an observational cohort study. Am J Sports Med 2010;38:1110–6.
95. Dave LY, Nyland J, McKee PB, et al. Mesenchymal stem cell therapy in the sports knee: where are we in 2011? Sports Health 2012;4:252–7.
96. Minas T, Gomoll AH, Solhpour S, et al. Autologous chondrocyte implantation for joint preservation in patients with early osteoarthritis. Clin Orthop Relat Res 2010;468:147–57.
97. Ghivizzani SC, Muzzonigro TS, Kang R, et al. Clinical gene therapy for arthritis. Drugs Today (Barc) 1999;35:389–96.
98. Ha CW, Noh MJ, Choi KB, et al. Initial phase I safety of retrovirally transduced human chondrocytes expressing transforming growth factor-beta-1 in degenerative arthritis patients. Cytotherapy 2012;14:247–56.

99. Hsieh JL, Shen PC, Shiau AL, et al. Intraarticular gene transfer of thrombospondin-1 suppresses the disease progression of experimental osteoarthritis. J Orthop Res 2010;28:1300–6.

100. Watson RS, Gouze E, Levings PP, et al. Gene delivery of TGF-beta1 induces arthrofibrosis and chondrometaplasia of synovium in vivo. Lab Invest 2010;90: 1615–27.

101. Terkeltaub R, Lotz M, Johnson K, et al. Parathyroid hormone-related proteins is abundant in osteoarthritic cartilage, and the parathyroid hormone-related protein 1-173 isoform is selectively induced by transforming growth factor beta in articular chondrocytes and suppresses generation of extracellular inorganic pyrophosphate. Arthritis Rheum 1998;41:2152–64.

102. Horie M, Choi H, Lee RH, et al. Intra-articular injection of human mesenchymal stem cells (MSCs) promote rat meniscal regeneration by being activated to express Indian hedgehog that enhances expression of type II collagen. Osteoarthr Cartil 2012;20:1197–207.

103. Davies MR, Ribeiro LR, Downey-Jones M, et al. Ligands for retinoic acid receptors are elevated in osteoarthritis and may contribute to pathologic processes in the osteoarthritic joint. Arthritis Rheum 2009;60:1722–32.

104. Ho LJ, Lin LC, Hung LF, et al. Retinoic acid blocks pro-inflammatory cytokine-induced matrix metalloproteinase production by down-regulating JNK-AP-1 signaling in human chondrocytes. Biochem Pharmacol 2005;70:200–8.

105. Saito S, Kondo S, Mishima S, et al. Analysis of cartilage-derived retinoic-acid-sensitive protein (CD-RAP) in synovial fluid from patients with osteoarthritis and rheumatoid arthritis. J Bone Joint Surg Br 2002;84:1066–9.

106. Li X, Peng J, Wu M, et al. BMP2 promotes chondrocyte proliferation via the Wnt/beta-catenin signaling pathway. Mol Med Rep 2011;4:621–6.

107. Yuasa T, Kondo N, Yasuhara R, et al. Transient activation of Wnt/{beta}-catenin signaling induces abnormal growth plate closure and articular cartilage thickening in postnatal mice. Am J Pathol 2009;175:1993–2003.

108. Song YW, Zhang T, Wang WB. Glucocorticoid could influence extracellular matrix synthesis through Sox9 via p38 MAPK pathway. Rheumatol Int 2012;32: 3669–73.

109. Kanazawa T, Furumatsu T, Hachioji M, et al. Mechanical stretch enhances COL2A1 expression on chromatin by inducing SOX9 nuclear translocalization in inner meniscus cells. J Orthop Res 2012;30:468–74.

110. Appleton CT, Usmani SE, Bernier SM, et al. Transforming growth factor alpha suppression of articular chondrocyte phenotype and Sox9 expression in a rat model of osteoarthritis. Arthritis Rheum 2007;56:3693–705.

111. Cucchiarini M, Thurn T, Weimer A, et al. Restoration of the extracellular matrix in human osteoarthritic articular cartilage by overexpression of the transcription factor SOX9. Arthritis Rheum 2007;56:158–67.

112. Gordon DF, Wagner J, Atkinson BL, et al. Human Cart-1: structural organization, chromosomal localization, and functional analysis of a cartilage-specific homeodomain cDNA. DNA Cell Biol 1996;15:531–41.

113. Zhao GQ, Eberspaecher H, Seldin MF, et al. The gene for the homeodomain-containing protein Cart-1 is expressed in cells that have a chondrogenic potential during embryonic development. Mech Dev 1994;48:245–54.

114. Kamekura S, Kawasaki Y, Hoshi K, et al. Contribution of runt-related transcription factor 2 to the pathogenesis of osteoarthritis in mice after induction of knee joint instability. Arthritis Rheum 2006;54:2462–70.

Index

Note: Page numbers of article titles are in **boldface** type.

Clin Sports Med 33 (2014) 175–179
http://dx.doi.org/10.1016/S0278-5919(13)00117-8
0278-5919/14/$ – see front matter © 2014 Elsevier Inc. All rights reserved.

sportsmed.theclinics.com

Moving?

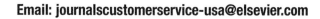

Make sure your subscription moves with you!

To notify us of your new address, find your **Clinics Account Number** (located on your mailing label above your name), and contact customer service at:

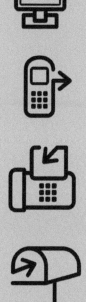

Email: journalscustomerservice-usa@elsevier.com

800-654-2452 (subscribers in the U.S. & Canada)
314-447-8871 (subscribers outside of the U.S. & Canada)

Fax number: 314-447-8029

Elsevier Health Sciences Division
Subscription Customer Service
3251 Riverport Lane
Maryland Heights, MO 63043

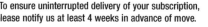

Printed and bound by CPI Group (UK) Ltd, Croydon, CR0 4YY

12/10/2024

01773480-0002